Teen Health Series

Stress Information For Teens,
Third Edition

Stress Information For Teens, Third Edition

Health Tips About The Mental And Physical Consequences Of Stress

Including Facts About The Causes Of Stress, Types Of Stressors, Effects Of Stress, Strategies For Managing Stress, And More

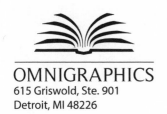

OMNIGRAPHICS
615 Griswold, Ste. 901
Detroit, MI 48226

Bibliographic Note
Because this page cannot legibly accommodate all the copyright notices, the Bibliographic Note portion of the
Preface constitutes an extension of the copyright notice.

* * *

OMNIGRAPHICS
Siva Ganesh Maharaja, *Managing Editor*

* * *

Copyright © 2018 Omnigraphics
ISBN 978-0-7808-1589-6
E-ISBN 978-0-7808-1590-2

Library of Congress Cataloging-in-Publication Data

Names: Omnigraphics, Inc., issuing body.

Title: Stress information for teens: health tips about the mental and physical consequences
of stress including information about the causes of stress, types of stressors, effects of stress,
strategies for managing stress, and more.

Description: Third edition. | Detroit, MI: Omnigraphics, Inc., [2017] | Series: Teen health series |
Audience: Grade 9 to 12. | Includes bibliographical references and index.

Identifiers: LCCN 2017041421 (print) | LCCN 2017042169 (ebook) | ISBN 9780780815902
(eBook) | ISBN 9780780815896 (hardcover: alk. paper)

Subjects: LCSH: Stress management for teenagers. | Stress (Psychology)

Classification: LCC RA785 (ebook) | LCC RA785.S766 2017 (print) | DDC 616.9/800835--dc23

LC record available at https://lccn.loc.gov/2017041421

Table Of Contents

Part Three: Effects Of Stress On The Body, Mind, And Behavior

Part Four: Diseases And Disorders With A Possible Stress Component

Part Five: Stress Management

Part Six: If You Need More Information

Preface

About This Book

Stress can be experienced not only by adults but also teens and children. Puberty's hormones can induce some especially confusing emotional and physical challenges in adolescents. The stresses teens feel can be good or bad. Some stress in response to internal or external pressures and expectations help teens to perform well and motivates them to do their best. On the other hand, unrealistic or overwhelming pressure stops being helpful, and it can have a negative impact on teens' health, mood, productivity, relationships, and behavior. Furthermore, stress left unchecked may result in emotional and physical consequences that can last a lifetime.

Stress Information For Teens, Third Edition helps readers understand what stress is, recognize the different types of stressors, and realize how stress affects the adolescent mind, body, and behavior. Common causes of teen stress are discussed, and diseases and disorders having possible stress components (including asthma, back pain, chronic fatigue, peptic ulcers, eczema, hair loss, and eating disorders) are explained. Facts about successful practices, therapies, and techniques for handling anger, improving body image and self-esteem, and relieving stress (such as exercise, relaxation techniques, massage therapy, meditation, yoga, art therapies, pet interaction, and journaling) are also included. The book concludes with a directory of stress and stress management resources and suggestions for additional reading.

How To Use This Book

This book is divided into parts and chapters. Parts focus on broad areas of interest; chapters are devoted to single topics within a part.

Part One: Understanding Stress examines stress and explains the distinctions between acute stress (short-term) and chronic stress (long-term). It explores stress in adolescents and discusses how suitable reactions to potentially stressful situations can actually help build resilience and self-esteem.

Part Two: Common Causes Of Stress In Teens includes information about the most frequent sources of stress among adolescents, including school, test anxiety, peer pressure, relationship and friendship issues, dating concerns, overbooked schedules, and sports competition. It also discusses stressors related to family life experiences (such as financial difficulty, violence, substance abuse, and divorce), current events, and social phobias. In addition, the causes and consequences of bullying—in person and online (cyberbullying)—are addressed.

Part Three: Effects Of Stress On The Body, Mind, And Behavior describes the various ways childhood stress can impact the entire lifespan. It discusses how stress affects the immune system, the potential link between stress and cancer, and how stress can change the brain—both physically and psychologically. Stress-related mental and behavioral disorders are addressed, including eating disorders, body dysmorphic disorder, self-injury, depression, and suicide. The special concerns associated with stresses related to loss and grief are also discussed.

Part Four: Diseases And Disorders With A Possible Stress Component explores how some illness and other health issues might be stress related. Chapters with information on medical conditions linked to stress triggers, such as asthma, chronic fatigue syndrome, fibromyalgia, multiple sclerosis, lupus, peptic ulcers, acid reflux, ulcerative colitis, and bowel syndromes, are included. Also, physical manifestations of chronic stress, including back pain, eczema, and hair loss, are discussed.

Part Five: Stress Management provides information on stress management and stress reduction techniques, including exercise, yoga, tai chi, meditation, and relaxation. It discusses how laughter, spirituality, journaling, pets, and art therapies can be used to help relieve stress and how talking to parents, therapists, and other adults has the potential to offer additional health benefits. In addition, the importance of self-esteem and anger management is addressed.

Part Six: If You Need More Information includes a directory of organizations and suggestions for additional reading to provide further materials about adolescent stress and stress management.

Bibliographic Note

This volume contains documents and excerpts from publications issued by the following government agencies: Centers for Disease Control and Prevention (CDC); Child Welfare Information Gateway; Federal Deposit Insurance Corporation (FDIC); Federal Occupational Health (FOH); National Aeronautics and Space Administration (NASA); National Cancer Institute (NCI); National Center for Complementary and Integrative Health (NCCIH); National Institute of Arthritis and Musculoskeletal and Skin Diseases (NIAMS); National Institute of Diabetes and Digestive and Kidney Diseases (NIDDK); National Institute of Mental Health (NIMH); National Institute of Neurological Disorders and Stroke (NINDS); National Institute on Alcohol Abuse and Alcoholism (NIAAA); National Institutes of Health (NIH); Office of Disease Prevention and Health Promotion (ODPHP); Office on Women's

Health (OWH); Substance Abuse and Mental Health Services Administration (SAMHSA); U.S. Department of Health and Human Services (HHS); and U.S. Department of Veterans Affairs (VA).

It may also contain original material produced by Omnigraphics and reviewed by medical consultants.

The photograph on the front cover is © Antonio Guillem/Shutterstock.

Medical Review

Omnigraphics contracts with a team of qualified, senior medical professionals who serve as medical consultants for the *Teen Health Series*. As necessary, medical consultants review reprinted and originally written material for currency and accuracy. Citations including the phrase, Reviewed (month, year)" indicate material reviewed by this team. Medical consultation services are provided to the *Teen Health Series* editors by:

Dr. Vijayalakshmi, MBBS, DGO, MD
Dr. Senthil Selvan, MBBS, DCH, MD
Dr. K. Sivanandham, MBBS, DCH, MS (Research), PhD

About The *Teen Health Series*

At the request of librarians serving today's young adults, the *Teen Health Series* was developed as a specially focused set of volumes within Omnigraphics' *Health Reference Series*. Each volume deals comprehensively with a topic selected according to the needs and interests of people in middle school and high school. Teens seeking preventive guidance, information about disease warning signs, medical statistics, and risk factors for health problems will find answers to their questions in the *Teen Health Series*. The *Series*, however, is not intended to serve as a tool for diagnosing illness, in prescribing treatments, or as a substitute for the physician/patient relationship. All people concerned about medical symptoms or the possibility of disease are encouraged to seek professional care from an appropriate healthcare provider.

If there is a topic you would like to see addressed in a future volume of the *Teen Health Series*, please write to:

Editor
Teen Health Series
Omnigraphics
615 Griswold, Ste. 901
Detroit, MI 48226

A Note About Spelling And Style

Teen Health Series editors use *Stedman's Medical Dictionary* as an authority for questions related to the spelling of medical terms and the *Chicago Manual of Style* for questions related to grammatical structures, punctuation, and other editorial concerns. Consistent adherence is not always possible, however, because the individual volumes within the *Series* include many documents from a wide variety of different producers and copyright holders, and the editor's primary goal is to present material from each source as accurately as is possible following the terms specified by each document's producer. This sometimes means that information in different chapters may follow other guidelines and alternate spelling authorities. For example, occasionally a copyright holder may require that eponymous terms be shown in possessive forms (Crohn's disease vs. Crohn disease) or that British spelling norms be retained (leukaemia vs. leukemia).

Part One
Understanding Stress

Chapter 1

What Is Stress?

Stress is a physical and emotional reaction that people experience as they encounter changes in life. Stress is a normal feeling. However, long-term stress may contribute to or worsen a range of health problems including digestive disorders, headaches, sleep disorders, and other symptoms. Stress may worsen asthma and has been linked to depression, anxiety, and other mental illnesses.

> The body responds to stress by releasing stress hormones. These hormones make blood pressure, heart rate, and blood sugar levels go up. Long-term stress can help cause a variety of health problems, including:
>
> - Mental health disorders, like depression and anxiety
> - Obesity
> - Heart disease
> - High blood pressure
> - Abnormal heart beats
> - Menstrual problems
> - Acne and other skin problems
>
> *(Source: "Stress And Your Health," National Women's Health Information Center (NWHIC), Office on Women's Health (OWH).)*

About This Chapter: Text in this chapter begins with excerpts from "Stress," National Center for Complementary and Integrative Health (NCCIH), February 27, 2017; Text under the heading "Five Things You Should Know About Stress" is excerpted from "5 Things You Should Know About Stress," National Institute of Mental Health (NIMH), December 20, 2016.

Some people use relaxation techniques (also called relaxation response techniques) to release tension and to counteract the ill effects of stress. Relaxation techniques often combine breathing and focused attention on pleasing thoughts and images to calm the mind and the body. Some examples of relaxation response techniques are autogenic training, biofeedback, deep breathing, guided imagery, progressive relaxation, and self-hypnosis. Mind and body practices, such as meditation and yoga, are also sometimes considered relaxation techniques.

Five Things You Should Know About Stress

1. **Stress affects everyone.** Everyone feels stressed from time to time. Some people may cope with stress more effectively or recover from stressful events more quickly than others. There are different types of stress—all of which carry physical and mental health risks. A stressor may be a one time or short-term occurrence, or it can be an occurrence that keeps happening over a long period of time.

   Examples of stress include:

   • Routine stress related to the pressures of work, school, family and other daily responsibilities

   • Stress brought about by a sudden negative change, such as losing a job, divorce, or illness

   • Traumatic stress experienced in an event like a major accident, war, assault, or a natural disaster where people may be in danger of being seriously hurt or killed. People who experience traumatic stress often experience temporary symptoms of mental illness, but most recover naturally soon after.

2. **Not all stress is bad.** Stress can motivate people to prepare or perform, like when they need to take a test or interview for a new job. Stress can even be life-saving in some situations. In response to danger, your body prepares to face a threat or flee to safety. In these situations, your pulse quickens, you breathe faster, your muscles tense, your brain uses more oxygen and increases activity—all functions aimed at survival.

3. **Long-term stress can harm your health.** Health problems can occur if the stress response goes on for too long or becomes chronic, such as when the source of stress is constant, or if the response continues after the danger has subsided. With chronic stress, those same life-saving responses in your body can suppress immune, digestive, sleep, and reproductive systems, which may cause them to stop working normally.

Different people may feel stress in different ways. For example, some people experience mainly digestive symptoms, while others may have headaches, sleeplessness, sadness, anger or irritability. People under chronic stress are prone to more frequent and severe viral infections, such as the flu or common cold.

Routine stress may be the hardest type of stress to notice at first. Because the source of stress tends to be more constant than in cases of acute or traumatic stress, the body gets no clear signal to return to normal functioning. Over time, continued strain on your body from routine stress may contribute to serious health problems, such as heart disease, high blood pressure, diabetes, and other illnesses, as well as mental disorders like depression or anxiety.

4. **There are ways to manage stress.** The effects of stress tend to build up over time. Taking practical steps to manage your stress can reduce or prevent these effects. The following are some tips that may help you to cope with stress:

    *   **Recognize the signs** of your body's response to stress, such as difficulty sleeping, increased alcohol and other substance use, being easily angered, feeling depressed, and having low energy.

    *   **Talk to your doctor or healthcare provider.** Get proper healthcare for existing or new health problems.

    *   **Get regular exercise.** Just 30 minutes per day of walking can help boost your mood and reduce stress.

    *   **Try a relaxing activity.** Explore stress coping programs, which may incorporate meditation, yoga, tai chi, or other gentle exercises. For some stress-related conditions, these approaches are used in addition to other forms of treatment. Schedule regular times for these and other healthy and relaxing activities.

    *   **Set goals and priorities.** Decide what must get done and what can wait, and learn to say no to new tasks if they are putting you into overload. Note what you have accomplished at the end of the day, not what you have been unable to do.

    *   **Stay connected** with people who can provide emotional and other support. To reduce stress, ask for help from friends, family, and community or religious organizations.

    *   **Consider a Clinical Trial.** Researchers at the National Institute of Mental Health (NIMH), National Center for Complementary and Integrative Health (NCCIH), and other research facilities across the country are studying the causes and effects of psychological stress, and stress management techniques.

5. **If you're overwhelmed by stress, ask for help from a health professional.** You should seek help right away if you have suicidal thoughts, are overwhelmed, feel you cannot cope, or are using drugs or alcohol to cope. Your doctor may be able to provide a recommendation.

Anyone experiencing severe or long-term, unrelenting stress can become overwhelmed. If you or a loved one is having thoughts of suicide, call the toll-free National Suicide Prevention Lifeline (NSPL) at 800-273-8255 (800-273-TALK), available 24 hours a day, 7 days a week. The service is available to anyone. All calls are confidential.

Chapter 2

Short- And Long-Term Stress

What Is Short-Term Stress?

Have you ever started a new school, argued with your best friend, or moved? Do you have to deal with the ups and downs of daily life—like homework or your parents' expectations? Then you already know about stress. In fact, everyone experiences stress. Your body is pre-wired to deal with it—whether it is expected or not. This response is known as the stress response, or fight or flight.

The fight or flight response is as old as the hills. In fact, when people used to have to fight off wild animals to survive, fight or flight is what helped them do it. Today, different things cause stress (when was the last time you had to fend off a grizzly bear?), but we still go through fight or flight. It prepares us for quick action—which is why the feeling goes away once whatever was stressing you out passes! It can also happen when something major happens—like if you change schools or have a death in your family.

Everyone has weird feelings when they are stressed. Fight or flight can cause things like sweaty palms or a dry mouth when you are nervous, or knots in your stomach after an argument with someone. This is totally normal and means that your body is working exactly like it should. There are lots of signs of stress—common types are physical (butterflies in your stomach), emotional (feeling sad or worried), behavioral (you don't feel like doing things), and mental (you can't concentrate). Most physical signs of stress usually don't last that long and can help you perform better, if you manage them right.

About This Chapter: This chapter includes text excerpted from "BAM! Body And Mind—Got Butterflies? Find Out Why," Centers for Disease Control and Prevention (CDC), May 9, 2015.

So, when you feel stress, what happens to make your body do the things it does? According to the experts, three glands "go into gear" and work together to help you cope with change or a stressful situation. Two are in your brain and are called the hypothalamus and the pituitary gland. The third, the adrenal glands, are on top of your kidneys. The hypothalamus signals your pituitary gland that it is time to tell your adrenal glands to release the stress hormones called epinephrine, norepinenphrine, and cortisol.

These chemicals increase your heart rate and breathing and provide a burst of energy—which is useful if you're trying to run away from a bear! These chemicals can also control body temperature (which can make you feel hot or cold), keep you from getting hungry, and make you less sensitive to pain. Because everyone is different, everyone will have different signs. Not to worry—everyone experiences these physical signs of stress sometimes. The good news is that, once things return to normal, your body will turn off the stress response. After some rest and relaxation, you'll be good as new.

Examples Of Short-Term Stress

You're about to take a big test or star in the school play and you've got cold hands, a mouth as dry as the desert, and your heart is pounding.

Cold Hands

Because you're nervous and under pressure to perform, your body has kicked the stress response into high gear. The stress hormones are shooting through your bloodstream and moving your blood away from your skin. This can give your heart and muscles more strength—which you would really need if you were trying to run away. Because your blood is going to the places that really need it (like your heart, lungs, and liver), your hands can be left feeling like ice.

Dry Mouth

Once that stress response is running full force, your body sends your blood to only those parts that are truly necessary for you to survive. Lots of the fluid in your body go to really important places (like your organs) and can leave you with a mouth as dry as the desert. Because your blood is busy with your organs and not your muscles, your throat (which is made of muscle) can tighten, making it hard to swallow.

Pounding Heart

When you're starring in the school play, your body wants to give you what you need to succeed—which goes back to the fight or flight response. Your heart will start pounding to help you out! In fact, it is one of the first signs of the stress response. It happens because the release of stress hormones can speed up the flow of your blood by 300–400 percent! Your heart has to beat much faster to move all of that blood to your organs and your muscles. This provides a burst of energy that can help you get through backstage jitters and the first few minutes of your play.

Everyone experiences stress. If you have any of these signs of stress, it means that your body is doing its job. Try to relax and check this out for some easy ways to cope with stress.

Red Face/Lots Of Sweat

- You're about to make an election speech for student council and your face is beet red, and you are sweaty all over.

Even though it's just a speech and you aren't planning on fighting off any tigers, remember what you are feeling is part of the fight or flight response. The body turns on its climate control system, raises its temperature, and produces sweat—and lots of it. Originally, this helped your body cool in case you did need to run away from a horde of wild animals. Of course, now that you are making your speech (which is the modern day equivalent of facing down those tigers and bears), you end up drenched in sweat and your face is the color of a fire engine.

Butterflies/Knots

- It's your first day back at school, or maybe you're starting a new school, and you've got butterflies in your stomach.

Stomachaches, or a queasy feeling, happen all the time in stressful situations like this. And it's no wonder. Once the stress response kicks into high gear, one of the stress hormones (cortisol) shuts the stomach down and won't let food digest. It can also put your digestive tract into high speed, making you feel nauseated.

Can't Concentrate?

- You have so much to do, but you just can't seem to concentrate.

Got too much to do? You know how it goes—you have tons of homework to do RIGHT NOW, you've got a game this afternoon, your little brother is annoying you, and your mom is insisting that you clean your room—but you just can't seem to focus on any one thing. You feel like you have no energy to finish all that you've got to do. This is because the stress hormones fill up your short-term memory with the immediate demands of dealing with stress. They also signal your brain to store the memory of the stressful event in your long-term memory so you know how to respond the next time something stressful happens. All of this means you are more likely to forget something, feel like you can't concentrate, snap at your family, be mean to a friend, or feel tongue-tied.

Common causes of short-term stress:

- Needing to do a lot in a short amount of time
- Experiencing many small problems in the same day, like a traffic jam or running late
- Getting lost
- Having an argument

Common causes of long-term stress:

- Problems at work or at home
- Money problems
- Caring for someone with a serious illness
- Chronic (ongoing) illness
- Death of a loved one

(Source: "Manage Stress," Office of Disease Prevention and Health Promotion (ODPHP), U.S. Department of Health and Human Services (HHS).)

What Is Long-Term Stress?

But what happens when life continues to throw curves at you and if you have one stressful event after another? Your stress response may not be able to stop itself from running overtime, and you may not have a chance to rest, restore, and recuperate. This can add up and, suddenly, the signs of overload hit you—turning short-term stressors into long-term stress. This means that you may have even more physical signs of stress. Things like a headache, eating too much or not at all, tossing and turning all night, or feeling down and angry all the time, are all signs of long-term stress. These signs start when you just can't deal with any more.

Long-term stress can affect your health and how you feel about yourself, so it is important to learn to deal with it. No one is completely free of stress and different people respond to it in lots of different ways. The most important thing to learn about long-term stress is how to spot it. You can do that by listening to your body signals and learning healthy ways to handle it.

Change In Appetite

You've just had a fight with your best friend and eating is the only thing that makes you feel better. Or, maybe you feel like you could never eat again.

While you might feel starved after a stressful event, your best friend might be grossed out by the thought of food. It just depends on how your body reacts to stress. If you get hungry, you may crave comfort foods (like chocolate, soda, or ice cream) because they increase the levels of a feel-good hormone called serotonin in the body. That means you probably will be in a better mood. Keep in mind that your body is just responding to the stress you are feeling. Your appetite will go back to normal.

On the other hand, your best friend might lose her appetite because the stress hormones make it difficult for her to eat. If you can't eat when you are stressed, try something small—like peanut butter toast or a piece of fruit.

Anger

Things are crazy right now and you just don't have any patience with anyone. You feel angry at the drop of a hat.

Anger is a common response to stress. Often, people who have been locked into a stress cycle feel helpless and overwhelmed. Once this happens, they can get angry much more quickly and they lash out at anyone that gets in their way. In fact, everyone at one point or another gets angry because they are stressed out.

Sleeplessness

You're exhausted but when you try to sleep, you lie awake for hours.

During the day, the levels of hormones that give you energy (epinephrine and norepinephrine) and those that help you stay happy (called dopamine) stay consistent. Towards the end of a normal day, these hormones begin to decrease and the hormone that helps you sleep (called serotonin) kicks into high gear. But if you've been trapped in a stress cycle, your body continues to produce those stress hormones from the adrenal glands. They "rev" up your body and block out the serotonin, making it hard to sleep even if you feel tired.

Overwhelmed

You are starting to feel overwhelmed by it all and you don't know if you can handle it.

Everyone has different ideas of what you should be doing. Sometimes it feels like you have so many different roles to play—good student, kid brother, sister, and friend—that things can seem out of control. It can make you tired just thinking about all you have to do! If you are feeling overwhelmed, you may notice that you can't sleep—which makes you cranky. Then, you realize that you don't feel like doing the things you like to do. You even might feel a little bit sad or anxious. You may begin to feel achy and tired all over. These are signs of being stressed out. Your stress response system is having a hard time turning off. Don't panic—your body is just trying to tell you something. Take the time to figure out what is stressing you out and try to reduce the load you're carrying.

Headache

It's been a long, tense day and you feel like you've got a rubber band squeezing around your head that just won't stop.

Headaches are one of the most common signs of long-term stress. They can feel dull and achy—just like a rubber band tightening around your head. Although it is unclear what exactly causes these headaches, tight head and neck muscles are generally thought to be to blame. The chemical messengers in your brain get really busy and tell your blood vessels to get really small. This means that less blood is getting to your head—and that can cause a headache. Your eyes, forehead, or the top of your head will be the first places you feel the pain.

Chapter 3

Adolescents And Stress

Teen Brain More Vulnerable To Stress

Teen brains rely on early-maturing brain structures that process fear differently than adult brains, according to an National Institute of Mental Health (NIMH)-funded study. As a result, teens may have more difficulty than adults in differentiating between danger and safety, leading to more pervasive stress and anxiety.

The Study

Things that frighten children or teens generally no longer frighten them as adults. So how does the adult brain distinguish between danger and safety, and what does the developing brain do differently?

To explore these questions, Jennifer Lau, Ph.D., of Oxford University (formerly at NIMH), and colleagues compared the brain activity of healthy youth with healthy adults during a threat learning task. In this task, participants were shown a series of photos that showed:

- A person with a neutral expression at first, then a fearful expression paired with a loud scream; or, in some later photos, the same person with a neutral expression only (threat stimulus)

- A different person with a neutral expression only (safety stimulus)

Immediately after each photo, participants rated how afraid they felt.

About This Chapter: This chapter includes text excerpted from "Teen Brain Less Discerning Of Threat Vs. Safety, More Vulnerable To Stress," National Institute of Mental Health (NIMH), April 28, 2011. Reviewed October 2017.

Teens And Stress

Stressing out about a boyfriend or girlfriend or history test is part of a typical day for a teenager. But what is making these insignificant events seem like the end of the world?

With help from the National Science Foundation (NSF), Adriana Galván, a psychologist at the University of California, Los Angeles (UCLA), has been studying the effects of stress on teenagers and adults.

"Teenagers experience stress as more stressful," says Galván, "and if that stress is interfering with their decision making, it's really important to understand the neural mechanism that's underlying this connection between high levels of stress and poor decision making."

Galván's ground-breaking study focuses on the effect stress has on brain function. Study participants report their stress level daily, using a one to seven scale—seven being the worst. If participants rate their day as a seven, Galván will ask them to visit the lab for tests.

Nilufer Rustomji, an 18-year-old participant of the study, rates her day's stress level as a seven. Monitoring her brain function with Magnetic Resonance Imaging (MRI), Galván asks Rustomji to play a simple "reward and risk" video game, which involves wagering money.

"During the game, Rustomji is evaluating risk," explains Galván, "and while she's doing that evaluation, we are taking pictures of the brain to see how the brain makes [such] risky choices."

After computer processing the images, Galván analyzes how stress and risk influence what she calls the "reward system."

"The teenagers show more activation in the reward system than adults when making risky choices, and they are also making more risky choices than adults are," says Galván.

The prefrontal cortex is the part of the brain that helps regulate behavior but in adolescents, this region is not fully developed.

To help lower teens' stress, Galván says teens should double check and think about how the consequences will affect them later. "When you are stressed out as a teenager, it's interfering with your ability to make decisions," says Galván. "It's interfering with how the brain functions in regions that are still developing, mainly the reward system and the prefrontal cortex."

Galván's study is helping to provide deeper insight into why teenagers often act the way they do.

(Source: "Teens And Stress," National Science Foundation (NSF).)

Results Of The Study

Both adults and teens reported feeling more afraid of the threat stimulus than the safety stimulus. Compared to adults, teens were less able to differentiate the threat from the safety stimulus.

Using functional magnetic resonance imaging, the researchers found that teens also had more activity in the hippocampus and right side of the amygdala than adults when viewing the threat stimulus compared with the safety stimulus. The hippocampus helps create and file new memories, while the amygdala activates the "fight-or-flight" response to stress and may be involved in fear learning.

Activity in another brain structure, the late-maturing dorsolateral prefrontal cortex (DLPFC), also differed between adults and teens. The DLPFC is highly involved in categorizing objects into different groups. In adults, activity increased as they rated more fear in relation to the safety stimulus. The researchers noted that this finding suggests that the adults' brains recruited the DLPFC more when they were unsure if a stimulus was safe or not safe. This uncertainty was reflected in their fear ratings.

Significance

The findings suggest that teen brains rely primarily on the hippocampus and right amygdala, brain structures that mature earlier in development and which are responsible for basic fear responses. In contrast, adults show more focused brain activity in prefrontal regions, which mature later in development. These regions are also involved in making more reasoned judgments about what is actually dangerous from what is safe.

According to the researchers, this difference may help to explain why teens generally report more pervasive worries and are more vulnerable to stress-related problems.

Chapter 4

Personality And Stress

The stress response, sometimes known as the "fight-or-flight" response, mobilizes the body's reserves to overcome a perceived threat. It evolved to protect people from danger and is considered essential to survival. When confronted with a stressful situation, the body increases its production of the chemicals cortisol, adrenaline, and noradrenaline. These chemicals trigger a faster heart rate, rapid breathing, muscle tension, and alertness. At the same time, the chemicals slow down nonessential body functions, such as the digestive and immune systems.

Taking Stock: My Body's Reaction To Stress

This is how a cat responds to stress. He turns sideways so he looks bigger. He fluffs out his fur and his tail so he looks bigger still. He bares his teeth. All these signs show that he's ready to fight. And if the cat doesn't fight, he's ready to flee—to run away from danger. Cats really do have a physical reaction to stress. It's called the "fight or flight" response. Believe it or not, people have this response, too. This response passed to use from our ancestors, who faced predators.

(Source: "The Body-Mind Connection Of Stress," Centers for Disease Control and Prevention (CDC).)

Stress can broadly be classified as physiological or psychological. Physiological stress refers to the adaptive mechanisms the body uses to respond to physical challenges, such as a broken bone or exposure to extreme cold. Psychological stress, on the other hand, refers to a disparity between an external stressor and the person's mental, emotional, or social resources. Examples might include feelings of anxiety about an upcoming test or worry about meeting a work deadline.

About This Chapter: "Personality And Stress," © 2018 Omnigraphics. Reviewed October 2017.

Even though the sources of psychological stress may not be life threatening, the body responds to them in much the same way as it responds to physiological stressors. These responses, while designed to protect the body, can actually have harmful effects on both physical and mental health when they recur frequently over prolonged periods of time. Chronic stress has been linked to a multitude of health conditions, including depression, digestive problems, fatigue, headaches, heart disease, high blood pressure, insomnia, muscle aches, and obesity.

Personality Types

- The response to stress is a complex and highly personalized mechanism involving many interrelated biological, psychological, and social factors. Studies have shown that an individual's personality—as determined by inherited characteristics, life experiences, and cognitive predispositions—strongly influences how they interpret and deal with stressful situations. People who demonstrate certain personality traits, such as resilience and adaptability, tend to respond better to adversity and be less susceptible to stress.

- Researchers have developed the Five Factor Model as a way to classify different personality types. The "Big Five" personality characteristics in this model include:

  - Openness to new experiences, as opposed to closed-mindedness

  - Conscientiousness, as opposed to disorganization

  - Extraversion, as opposed to introversion

  - Agreeableness, as opposed to disagreeableness

  - Neuroticism, as opposed to emotional stability

Although age, gender, intellect, and other factors can influence a person's sensitivity to stressors, studies have shown that personality type is an important factor in determining an individual's reaction to stress. In fact, personality traits can help explain how some people can handle huge amounts of stress for long periods of time, while others may feel overwhelmed when faced with small amounts of stress on a temporary basis.

An individual's personality influences every stage of the stress response, from evaluating whether or not a situation is stressful to choosing coping methods. In general, individuals with strong scores in extraversion tend to be optimistic and develop good problem-solving and coping strategies. They can reappraise potentially stressful situations in a positive way—for instance, as a challenge and an opportunity for growth and personal development—and effectively seek social support to help them deal with the stressor. On the other hand, individuals with strong scores in neuroticism tend to be pessimistic. They can become overwhelmed by potentially stressful situations, which can take a toll on their life satisfaction and physical health.

Type A And Type B Behavior

The theory of Type A behavior was developed in the 1950s by American cardiologist Meyer Friedman, who noticed a link between a certain personality type and the risk of heart disease. His 1974 book on the theory opened up a new field of research that looked beyond the well-known risk factors of diet and cholesterol and examined the mind-body connection to heart disease. The term "Type A personality" soon became a national buzzword to refer to high-stress personalities who tended to be driven, impatient, and competitive. This personality type was considered to be in opposition to Type B personalities, who tended to be calm, steady, relaxed, and less vulnerable to stress.

Type A personalities are believed to have an overactive sympathetic nervous system pathway. This pathway is responsible for stimulating the "fight-or-flight" response, which is associated with increased secretions of the emergency hormones that elevate the heart and respiratory rates and may contribute to hypertension and heart disease. In Type B personalities, the parasympathetic nervous system pathway is dominant. This pathway is associated with a lower metabolic rate and the release of "feel-good" neurotransmitters like endorphin, melatonin, and serotonin.

Critics argue, however, that human behavior is too complex to be categorized within the narrow parameters outlined by Friedman. Modern-day psychologists generally refrain from drawing a clear distinction between the two extreme personality types, preferring to regard them as points on a continuum. In addition, some psychologists argue that personality and experiences do not necessarily condition people to respond to stress in a certain way. Instead, they claim that people can learn to manage stress effectively through training programs that help them build self-confidence, develop problem-solving skills, and face the everyday challenges of life in a more positive manner.

Reference

McLeod, Saul. "Type A Personality." Simply Psychology, 2011.

Part Two
Common Causes Of Stress In Teens

Chapter 5

What Causes Stress In Kids

Adults assume that teens have nothing to stress about since their basic needs are being taken care of, and young people don't appear to have many responsibilities. Nothing could be further than the truth. Teens are, in fact, highly sensitive to changes around them and must deal with plenty of stress. Things that are not a big deal for adults often matter very much to younger people. Much of the stress that kids face is not harmful and may actually have some positive aspects. For example, a reasonable amount of stress can help teens prepare for a test, deliver a presentation, or perform better in a sports event. But if stress is intense and lingers for days on end, there are chances that it could have repercussions on the individual's health.

Teens often do not recognize that they are feeling stressed. Instead, they might feel they are sad, worried, confused, or angry. Using negative statements to describe themselves or the world around them could be a possible indicator that they're feeling stressed.

> Certain kinds of stress such as those imposed by teachers and coaches help kids stay motivated and keep up grades and athletic performance.

Some Causes Of Stress In Teens

Young people are under considerable pressure these days, including demands from school, family, activities, and friends. Teens can also set high standards for themselves and expect to meet those demands, as well. Stress can result when they are not able to live up to expectations. The following are some examples of stress in teens:

About This Chapter: "What Causes Stress In Kids," © 2018 Omnigraphics. Reviewed October 2017.

- Failure to meet the demands of parents, teachers, or coaches

- Peer pressure

- Self-imposed pressure

- Changing teachers

- Making friends and sustaining them

- Coping with a bully

- Feeling pressured to dress a certain way

- Failure to perform well in a sports event.

- Pressure to achieve high grades to get into a good college

- Moving to a new neighborhood

- Lack of enough free time

- Inability to overcome impairment

- Illness or death of a loved one

- Divorce in the family

- Observing parents worrying

- Concern about catastrophes or terrorism

Signs And Symptoms Of Stress

Teens can exhibit negative changes in behavior when they are stressed, and identifying them is a good first step in beginning to deal with the issue. Here are a few examples of stress-related changes:

- Loss of appetite

- Overeating

- Change in sleep patterns

- Bedwetting

- Becoming irritable or moody

- Frequently talking about being worried

- Being surprised or fearful

- Having nightmares

- Frequent crying

- Avoiding school

- Leaving friends and joining a new peer group

- Defying authority

- Being hostile or clingy with parents

- Bullying others

- A drop in academic performance

- Having an abundance of physical complaints

Reducing Stress

Teens with an easy-going temperament generally are able to negotiate daily hassles and problems successfully. They adapt to new circumstances and adjust to events easily. But some kids get thrown off balance in these types of situations. The ability to handle stress largely depends on whether individuals have had experience successfully handling challenges in the past and have the support of family members. Young people who feel they are competent, loved, and supported generally tend to handle stress better.

It is important to take care of your body by eating nutritious food, getting plenty of rest, and exercising regularly to counter stress. Parents can help their teens reduce stress by spending time with them, being available, and supporting them. Taking an interest in the teen's activities can help them feel that they are being held in regard. Parents can talk to their teens about what is causing stress and help think of solutions to problems that may be leading to it. For instance, if teens are engaged in too many activities after school, it might make sense to discuss which could be eliminated or curtailed.

Parents and teens could work together to develop strategies for situations like being bullied, such as walking away or contacting an adult who is charge. Some teens might benefit from relaxation techniques, such as breathing exercises, to reduce stress. They can also take their minds off of stress by indulging in a variety of activities or hobbies, like drawing or painting.

Why Teens Are Increasingly Stressed Out

Change in family dynamics is one of the biggest contributors to stress in teens. Young people of this generation tend to be more stressed out than the previous ones, and they seem to have fewer avenues of social support. Families in the past were frequently larger, so kids had the support of an extended family, including grandparents, aunts, and uncles. Such family structures have become a rarity today. On top of this, the incidence of divorce and fractured families has increased since most parents were teens. It is important for parents to pause their own work and activities on a regular basis to make time for their teens. They need to combat stress for both themselves and their children amidst their hectic lives.

> A breakdown of family structures that existed in older generations may have contributed to increasing incidence of stress in teens.

References

1. Dowshen, Steven, MD. "Childhood Stress," The Nemours Foundation, February 2015.

2. "Identifying Signs of Stress in Your Children and Teens," American Psychological Association, n.d.

3. "Helping Children Handle Stress," American Academy of Pediatrics, November 21, 2015.

4. "Stress Management for Children and Adults," Stop Child Abuse Now (SCAN), n.d.

Chapter 6

Current Events And Stress: News You Can Use

The news can be full of stories about unexpected or bad things like tornadoes or hurricanes, disease threats, bombings, kidnappings, and war. And the scary thing is—it may seem like these things are happening all around you, even in places where you feel secure like school, the mall, and at home. Seeing these things on TV or even experiencing them first hand (like being in a tornado) can cause you to feel uncertain, worried, or scared. These feelings may last even after the event is over.

Here are some tips to understanding the news and what you see and hear:

- **The news doesn't talk about everyday activities.** Instead, the news talks about things that are out of the ordinary—both good and bad. And sometimes it seems like the news shows more of the bad stuff—things like tragedies and crime. For example, if a plane crashes, it will get a lot of attention in the news—so much so, that you may think planes crash all the time. But in fact, thousands of planes take off and land safely each day—the news just doesn't talk about it.

- **Sometimes you see stories over and over about tragic events like bombings, or disasters such as floods, earthquakes, or hurricanes.** This doesn't mean these things are happening all the time—it just means that the news is talking about it again. The news will cover something when it first happens and then repeat the story. So you may see it on the news when you get home from school and then again before you go to bed. After the first day, the news may do what is called a "follow-up" story to tell you what happened after the event. So you may hear about the same thing for a few days, even though it only happened once.

About This Chapter: This chapter includes text excerpted from "BAM! Body And Mind—News You Can Use," Centers for Disease Control and Prevention (CDC), May 9, 2015.

- **Bad things in the news can alert you to what is going on around you.** For example, a news story could tell you about someone in your community who is breaking into homes. While this may scare you, just remember that even though it's on the news, that doesn't mean it will happen to you. But stories like this can help make you aware of your surroundings and of things you can do to protect yourself (like locking your doors!).

- **Disasters or tragic events can bring out the best in people.** Firemen and policemen are doing their jobs (like saving people) and volunteers and everyday citizens also are there to help. You will see people in your community volunteering to bring food and clothing to help people who are affected, families coming together to help each other out, and shelters being put into place to give people a place to stay. You can get involved too!

- **It is normal to be concerned about what you hear in the news.** But it is important to know that while things may seem uncertain for a while, your life usually will return to normal fairly soon.

Weave Your Own Safety Net

Following these tips can help you get on with your day-to-day life, even during stressful times.

Talk to your friends and your family and spend time with them. If you find yourself feeling unsafe, uncertain, worried, or scared, or if you don't understand what is going on around you, talk to your parents, teachers, or a school counselor. Your parents or other adults can help explain these events so you can understand things better. By talking with your friends and your family, you can share your feelings and know you are not alone. Plus, spending time with them may help you feel more safe and secure.

Help out others. Sometimes when you are concerned about what is going on around you, it is helpful to give others support. You can help out by raising money, donating clothes, or organizing an event like a food drive at your school to collect food and/or supplies for an organization that helps people affected by war, terrorism, or natural disasters. Even if you and your family are the ones who are affected by a disaster, helping others can help you deal with your own stress—it may make you feel a little more in control.

Write your feelings down. Writing your feelings down—in a diary, a journal, or even on a piece of scrap paper—is a great way to get things off of your chest. You can write down how you feel, what's going on in your life, or anything else!

Stick to your normal routine. There is comfort in the little things you do every day—so keep on doing them! And take care of yourself. Get lots of sleep, eat well, and be physically active.

Take a break from the TV news—watch a funny movie, play some games, go outside and play, or read a funny book or magazine. Too much information about disasters can get you down, so change your pace and watch some cartoons, read a joke book, or even make up your own. Did you know that smiling has been proven to improve your mood? That can help you feel like new and take your mind off things for a while.

Plan Ahead

Sometimes things happen that we just can't anticipate. But a few things (like hurricanes, tornadoes, or forest fires) occur in certain areas of the country during certain seasons. If you live in areas where weather "can take you by storm," you can take a few steps to help prepare in case of an emergency. Being prepared can help you feel like you have more control in an emergency, and help you feel less stressed.

Make a plan. Talk to your parents about being prepared. Just like your family should have a plan to get out of the house in case of a fire, make a plan in case bad weather strikes. Choose a place to go, who you would call, or what you would do. Make sure to talk about what you should do if you are at school, or a friend's house, or if your parents are at work.

Have an emergency supply kit. During or after a storm, you may be without power for a few days or you may not be able to leave your home. Work with your parents to put together a supply kit for such emergencies. Some things to have on hand include water, and nonperishable (that means they won't spoil) foods such as crackers, peanut butter, and canned food (soup, fruit, veggies, etc.). Make sure to have a battery-powered radio, flashlights, and extra batteries on hand. A First-Aid kit, facial tissue and toilet paper are good things to consider packing. Lanterns (lamp oil) or candles for light are good things to have, too. Also, don't forget about your family pet. Pack extra water and food for your four-legged friends.

Put together an Activity Survival Kit. Having some favorite books and games on hand will keep you interested and help pass the time. And while you may not want to live without power forever, being without it for a few days may be fun—it could give you an idea of what life was like before electricity!

Chapter 7

Stress From Every Day Life

Youth stress is usually related to everyday experiences, worries and challenges at school, home, in the community and within their peer group. For example, young people may experience stress resulting from bullying, name calling, social isolation, not getting what they want, body image, academic difficulties, or unsafe neighborhoods.

While each youth will respond to and resolve stress differently, the impact of ongoing and/or unresolved stress can lead to feelings of anxiety, depression, irritability, poor concentration, aggression, physical illness, fatigue, sleep disturbance and poor coping skills such as tobacco, drug and/or alcohol use.

Stress is not all bad. Stress helps you to deal with life's challenges, to give your best performance, and to meet a tough situation with focus. The body's stress response is important and necessary. However, when too much stress builds up, you may encounter many physical and emotional health problems. If you don't deal with stress, the health problems can stay with you and worsen over the course of your life.

Therefore, young people, like adults, can benefit from learning and practicing stress management skills. Youths who develop stress reduction skills learn how to feel and cope better without hurting themselves, or others. Identifying and acknowledging the causes of stress and expressing feelings about them are usually the most effective tools youths have to reduce stress, in addition to learning practical stress reduction skills.

About This Chapter: Text in this chapter begins with excerpts from "Expeditionary Skills For Life—Cope With It," National Aeronautics and Space Administration (NASA), April 1, 2017; Text under the heading "Feelin' Frazzled? Totally Tense Under Pressure?" is excerpted from "BAM! Body And Mind—Your Life—Feelin' Frazzled," Centers for Disease Control and Prevention (CDC), May 9, 2015.

Feelin' Frazzled? Totally Tense Under Pressure?

Finding yourself in a hectic situation, whether it's forgetting your homework or missing your ride home, can really stress you out. Are you looking for a safety net for those days that seem to get worse by the second? Could you really use some advice on how to de-stress both your body and your mind? Knowing how to deal can be half the battle!

Check out these ten tips to keep you cool, calm, and collected:

1. **Put your body in motion.** Moving from the chair to the couch while watching TV is not being physically active! Physical activity is one of the most important ways to keep stress away by clearing your head and lifting your spirits. Physical activity also increases endorphin levels—the natural "feel-good" chemicals in the body which leave you with a naturally happy feeling.

   Whether you like full-fledged games of football, tennis, or roller hockey, or you prefer walks with family and friends, it's important to get up, get out, and get moving!

2. **Fuel up.** Start your day off with a full tank—eating breakfast will give you the energy you need to tackle the day. Eating regular meals (this means no skipping dinner) and taking time to enjoy them (nope, eating in the car on the way to practice doesn't count) will make you feel better too. Make sure to fuel up with fruits, vegetables, proteins (peanut butter, a chicken sandwich, or a tuna salad) and grains (wheat bread, pasta, or some crackers)—these will give you the power you need to make it through those hectic days.

   Don't be fooled by the jolt of energy you get from sodas and sugary snacks—this only lasts a short time, and once it wears off, you may feel sluggish and more tired than usual. For that extra boost of energy to sail through history notes, math class, and after school activities, grab a banana, some string cheese, or a granola bar for some power-packed energy!

3. **LOL!** Some say that laughter is the best medicine—well, in many cases, it is! Did you know that it takes 15 facial muscles to laugh? Lots of laughin' can make you feel good—and, that good feeling can stay with you even after the laughter stops. So, head off stress with regular doses of laughter by watching a funny movie or cartoons, reading a joke book (you may even learn some new jokes), or even make up your own riddles...laughter can make you feel like a new person!

Everyone has those days when they do something really silly or stupid—instead of getting upset with yourself, laugh out loud! No one's perfect! Life should be about having fun. So, lighten up!

4. **Have fun with friends.** Being with people you like is always a good way to ditch your stress. Get a group together to go to the movies, shoot some hoops, or play a board game—or just hang out and talk. Friends can help you work through your problems and let you see the brighter side of things.

5. **Spill to someone you trust.** Instead of keeping your feelings bottled up inside, talk to someone you trust or respect about what's bothering you. It could be a friend, a parent, someone in your family, or a teacher. Talking out your problems and seeing them from a different view might help you figure out ways to deal with them. Just remember, you don't have to go it alone!

6. **Take time to chill.** Pick a comfy spot to sit and read, daydream, or even take a snooze. Listen to your favorite music. Work on a relaxing project like putting together a puzzle or making jewelry.

    Stress can sometimes make you feel like a tight rubber band—stretched to the limit! If this happens, take a few deep breaths to help yourself unwind. If you're in the middle of an impossible homework problem, take a break! Finding time to relax after (and sometimes during) a hectic day or week can make all the difference.

7. **Catch some zzzzz...** Fatigue is a best friend to stress. When you don't get enough sleep, it's hard to deal—you may feel tired, cranky, or you may have trouble thinking clearly. When you're overtired, a problem may seem much bigger than it actually is. You may have a hard time doing a school assignment that usually seems easy, you don't do your best in sports or any physical activity, or you may have an argument with your friends over something really stupid.

    Sleep is a big deal! Getting the right amount of sleep is especially important for kids your age. Because your body (and mind) is changing and developing, it requires more sleep to recharge for the next day. So don't resist, hit the hay!

8. **Keep a journal.** If you're having one of those crazy days when nothing goes right, it's a good idea to write things down in a journal to get it off of your chest—like how you feel, what's going on in your life, and things you'd like to accomplish. You could even write down what you do when you're faced with a stressful situation, and then look

back and think about how you handled it later. So, find a quiet spot, grab a notebook and pen, and start writing!

9. **Get it together.** Too much to do but not enough time? Forgot your homework? Feeling overwhelmed or discombobulated? Being unprepared for school, practice, or other activities can make for a very stressful day! Getting everything done can be a challenge, but all you have to do is plan a little and get organized.

10. **Lend a hand.** Get involved in an activity that helps others. It's almost impossible to feel stressed out when you're helping someone else. It's also a great way to find out about yourself and the special qualities you never knew you had! Signing up for a service project is a good idea, but helping others is as easy as saying hello, holding a door, or volunteering to keep a neighbor's pet. If you want to get involved in a more organized volunteer program, try working at a local recreation center, or helping with an after school program. The feeling you will get from helping others is greater than you can imagine!

Most importantly, don't sweat the small stuff! Try to pick a few really important things and let the rest slide—getting worked up over every little thing will only increase your stress. So, toughen up and don't let stressful situations get to you! Remember, you're not alone—everyone has stresses in their lives…it's up to you to choose how to deal with them.

Chapter 8

Test Anxiety

What Is Test Anxiety?

Test anxiety occurs when a person is excessively apprehensive about taking a test. The condition causes distress that can negatively affect performance on the exam, sometimes making the individual forget what he or she previously learned. Someone with test anxiety might lose concentration, become tense, and completely lose focus.

It is normal to be apprehensive before a test, and being nervous can actually have some benefits. For example, a small degree of stress can help you get started on a task and keep you going until you complete it. And it can help you focus better and complete the task properly. But when facing a test, some people become overly nervous to the point where performance suffers, and they experience symptoms that make it difficult to concentrate. When teens have test anxiety their mental faculties may become clouded, and studies show that all kinds of students, regardless of age or ability, can be prone to this condition. Preparation might be affected by insufficient study, lack of time, difficult material, physical exhaustion, or lack of sleep the night before the test. The feeling that you have not prepared properly and will not perform well can result in the symptoms of test anxiety.

Test anxiety is a kind of performance anxiety. This is something that people often experience when they need to go on stage or do something in front of others. In such situations, there is pressure to do well, which creates a high level of anxiety. This is commonly seen when someone has to perform in a play, give a speech, appear for a job interview, or play in front of a crowd.

Performing poorly on a test because of personal issues or crises at home should not be confused with test anxiety. Some of these issues, such as the death of a close relative,

About This Chapter: "Text Anxiety," © 2018 Omnigraphics. Reviewed October 2017.

would naturally interfere with concentration in a test and would not be considered test anxiety.

What Are The Signs Of Text Anxiety?

Test anxiety affects you mentally and physically. If you have the condition, you could completely forget what you learned and have difficulty concentrating. You can become overwhelmed with negative thoughts about how you are going to complete the test and what will happen if you fail. You might also dwell on how others are performing on the test, imaging them having much less trouble than you.

Physically, people with test anxiety may feel a fluttering known as "butterflies" in their stomach, and might also experience sweating and shaking. They might have a tension headache or feel like fainting or throwing up. Other symptoms associated with the condition include nausea, cramps, dry mouth, muscle tension, and increased breathing and heart rates. These symptoms can have an additional negative impact on test preparation and performance.

What Causes Test Anxiety?

Typically, anxiety occurs when you anticipate something stressful. This is the result of an evolutionary mechanism built into human beings known as the "fight-or-flight" response. The body prepares either to defend itself or flee from a potential threat by releasing a hormone known as adrenaline. Adrenaline causes the physical symptoms associated with test anxiety, such as shaking, sweating, muscle tension, heavy breathing, and a pounding heart. Negative thoughts, such as thinking that you will forget the answers or fail the test, adds to the anxiety and creates a vicious cycle that further worsens performance.

Who Can Suffer From Text Anxiety?

Anyone can be overcome with test anxiety, but perfectionists tend to be most prone to the condition. For them anything less than a perfect score is unacceptable, and they can be extremely fearful of making mistakes. They put pressure on themselves to perform better, which in turn creates a perfect environment for test anxiety. For many people, failing to prepare well enough can lead to test anxiety.

How Can You Cope With Test Anxiety?

Most students with test anxiety worry that they are not smart enough or sufficiently prepared to succeed. Such a mindset can be paralyzing when taking tests. Students must overcome these thoughts and view themselves as competent learners to overcome test anxiety.

Below are some strategies that can help teens deal with test anxiety more effectively.

1. **Mental Preparation**

    Students can do several things to prepare themselves better, some of which are listed below.

    - Develop good study habits. There's much more to learning than just attending classes. It is impossible to prepare for a test just by sitting in a classroom. It's equally important to develop good study habits and review schedules.

    - Be thorough. Rather than just memorizing, concentrate on the major ideas, main events, and most important issues covered in the material. Avoid anxiety with a solid understanding of the subject matter.

    - Review the material. Go over what you've learned by covering it throughout the week. This helps in committing the material to memory.

    - Don't cram. It is not advisable to study hard just before the exam. You cannot digest an entire chapter or term in just one night. Plan your study routine in advance, and review accordingly to avoid last-minute tension.

    - Know the test format clearly in advance. Doing this takes the initial shock you might experience when you see the test for the first time.

    - Write out your own possible questions and answers before the test. This will help you master the topics and feel more prepared.

    - Don't think negatively. Negative thoughts can disrupt your study schedule. Always think about positive outcomes.

    - Don't expect perfection. You don't have to know everything about a topic or the answer to every possible question.

    - Arrive early. Be at the test location well ahead of the test starting time, so you have time to relax with your friends. And don't discuss the test material. Last minute reviews can only serve to confuse you.

2. **Planning**

    Having a strategy in place before you take the test can help reduce anxiety.

Some helpful strategies include the following:

- When the test paper is handed out, it is normal to feel tense. Once you have the paper in hand, take a few seconds to calm down before you start.

- Plan your time so you can answer all the questions. Allow more time for the most difficult questions. And don't dwell on any one question. Move on to the next item, and can come back to it later.

- If you are surprised by a question, don't lose your cool. Try answering something easy, and then come back after you've calmed down and can give it more time.

- If you felt confident answering a question the first time around, don't second-guess yourself and change the answer. This fosters negativity and could just be a waste of time.

- If you don't know the answer to a question, just accept that. If you feel the questions shouldn't have been on the test, you can discuss it with your teacher later.

3. Physical Preparation

It is important to take care of your health and pay attention to how you behave prior to a test in order to avoid anxiety-related problems. For example:

- Eat well. Adequate nutrition is an important part of studying before tests. Feeling weak and cranky during study time can lead to frustration and anxiety.

- Make time for physical activity. Exercising regularly helps you maintain a positive attitude. Do not disrupt your exercise schedule during test preparation.

- Get plenty of sleep. Lack of sleep affects memory and concentration. Staying up late studying and then getting up early can be counterproductive at exactly the wrong time.

- Socialize with friends and family and take regular breaks. Social interaction minimizes anxiety and helps reenergize you for additional study. Blend with people with a positive attitude. In particular, avoid those who think negatively, especially about tests.

- Don't procrastinate. If you put off your study schedule, you might be setting yourself up for cramming. And it's possible that you could be waiting until the last minute so you have an excuse for not doing well.

4. Relaxation Techniques

A number of relaxation techniques can help relieve anxiety, improve memory and enhance test performance.

Some suggestions:

- When you start to feel anxious, try deep breathing exercises. With your eyes closed, inhale slowly and deeply through your nose, and exhale very slowly through your mouth. Repeat until you feel yourself begin to feel less tense.

- Progressive muscle relaxation can help reduce stress. For example, contract your shoulders for ten seconds, then slowly loosen up and let your muscles relax. Repeat with hands, arms, legs, and feet. Concentrate on how the actions feel and try to become more relaxed with each repetition.

- Visualization exercises may help ease anxiety. Close your eyes and imagine yourself in a calm environment, such as a beach, a forest, or a spa. Combine this with a deep-breathing routine to increase the effect.

- If you regularly practice yoga, tai chi, or meditation, use these techniques to take a break from study. They can help you return to your work in a more relaxed frame of mind.

Being Successful

It takes time and practice to learn how to reduce test anxiety. A good attitude towards studying determines how well you perform on a test, so the best way to deal with test anxiety is to study well and be prepared in all respects. Since test anxiety thrives on the unknown, it is important to use good study techniques and learn the material thoroughly. When students feel confident of their knowledge and develop effective test-taking strategies, they can overcome test anxiety.

References

1. Ehmke, Rachel. "Tips For Beating Test Anxiety," Child Mind Institute, Inc.

2. Lyness, D'Arcy, PhD. "Test Anxiety," The Nemours Foundation, July, 2013.

3. "Reducing Test Anxiety," Educational Testing Service (ETS), n.d.

4. "Reducing Test Anxiety," Pittsburg State University, n.d.

Chapter 9

Peer Pressure

Your classmates keep asking you to have them over because you have a pool, everyone at school is wearing silly hats so you do too, and your best friend begs you to go running with her because you both need more exercise, so you go, too. These are all examples of peer pressure. Don't get it yet?

- Pressure is the feeling that you are being pushed toward making a certain choice—good or bad.

- A peer is someone in your own age group.

- Peer pressure is—you guessed it—the feeling that someone your own age is pushing you toward making a certain choice, good or bad.

Why Peer Pressure Can Work?

Have you ever given into pressure? Like when a friend begs to borrow something you don't want to give up or to do something your parents say is off limits? Chances are you probably have given into pressure at some time in your life.

How did it feel to give into pressure? If you did something you wish you hadn't, then most likely you didn't feel too good about it. You might have felt...

- sad

- anxious

- guilty

About This Chapter: This chapter includes text excerpted from "Peer Pressure," The Cool Spot, National Institute on Alcohol Abuse and Alcoholism (NIAAA), October 29, 2016.

- like a wimp or pushover

- disappointed in yourself

Everyone gives in to pressure at one time or another, but why do people sometimes do things that they really don't want to do? Here are a few reasons. They...

- are afraid of being rejected by others

- want to be liked and don't want to lose a friend

- want to appear grown up

- don't want to be made fun of

- don't want to hurt someone's feelings

- aren't sure of what they really want

- don't know how to get out of the situation

When you face pressure you can stand your ground.

How Peers Pressure?

Almost everyone faces peer pressure once in a while. Friends have a big influence on our lives, but sometimes they push us to do things that we may not want to do. Unless you want to give in every time you face this, you're going to need to learn how to handle it.

The first step to standing up to peer pressure is to understand it. In this section, you'll start by learning to recognize the different things people do when they pressure others. Check out the differences between spoken and unspoken pressures, and learn about the peer pressure bag of tricks.

Soon you'll be able to spot peer pressure and deal with it!

Spoken Versus Unspoken Pressure

Sometimes a friend can say something directly to you that puts a lot of pressure on you and makes it hard to say no. This is **spoken pressure**.

You may think you are supposed to act or dress a certain way because it seems like everyone else is doing it, or because it's the cool thing to do. When you feel this way even though nobody has said anything about it, this is **unspoken pressure**.

If you haven't already, you are going to face both spoken and unspoken pressure in the future. It's just part of life. The important part is to make the right choices when a peer pressure situation comes up.

Peer Pressure Bag Of Tricks

Who needs you as a friend anyway? You're such a baby! It won't hurt bad!

Have your friends ever used these lines on you? Did you give in, even though you didn't want to?

These are a few of the goodies in the Peer Pressure Bag-of-Tricks. The tricks include put-downs, rejections, and reasoning, as well as pressure without words, or unspoken pressure.

A lot of people are standing up for what they believe in these days. Sooner or later, you'll probably have the chance to do that, too. If you feel pressured into using drugs or anything else you don't want to do, you can resist.

The power to resist.

"Resist" means you don't give in to, or go along with, something that somebody wants you to do. Resisting peer pressure can be a challenge—especially for teens, who often want to impress their friends, even if it means taking a risk.

(Source: "Drugs And Health Blog—Resisting Peer Pressure," National Institute on Drug Abuse (NIDA) for Teens.)

The Tricks

Learn to spot the tricks. Being aware of the pressure is the first step to resisting it.

Rejection: Threatening to end a friendship or a relationship. This pressure can be hard to resist because nobody wants to lose friends. Some examples of pressure by rejection are:

- Who needs you as a friend anyway?

- If you don't drink we won't hang out any more.

- Why don't you leave if you don't want to drink with us?

Put downs: Insulting or calling a person names to make them feel bad. Some examples of put downs are:

- You're never any fun.

- You're such a baby.

- You're such a wimp.

- You're so uncool.

Reasoning: Telling a person reasons why they should try something or why it would be OK if they did. (Nobody said these were good reasons.) Some examples of pressure by reasoning are:

- It won't hurt you.

- Your parents will never find out.

- You'll have more fun.

Unspoken pressure: This is something you feel without anyone saying anything to you. You feel unspoken pressure if you want to do the same things others doing. Some unspoken pressure tricks are:

- The Huddle: A group of kids standing together in which everyone is talking and maybe looking at something you can't see, laughing and joking.

- The Look: Kids who think they're cool give you a certain look that means we're cool and you're not.

- The Example: A group of popular kids decide to get the same backpack and you want one too.

Peer Pressure Can Be Good, Too

Peer pressure isn't all bad. You and your friends can pressure each other into some things that will improve your health and social life and make you feel good about your decisions.

Think of a time when a friend pushed you to do something good for yourself or to avoid something that would've been bad.

Here are some good things friends can pressure each other to do:

- Be honest

- Avoid Alcohol

- Avoid drugs

- Not smoke

- Be nice

- Respect others

- Work hard

- Exercise (together!)

You and your friends can also use good peer pressure to help each other resist bad peer pressure.

If you see a friend taking some heat, try some of these lines...

- We don't want to drink.

- We don't need to drink to have fun.

- Let's go and do something else.

- Leave her alone. She said she didn't want any.

Chapter 10

Relationships: Friends And Dating

Friends

Friendships can be fantastic, but they also can be tough at times. The main thing to remember is that good friends support you, respect you, and like you for who you really are!

What Are True Friends?

True friends:

- Want you to be happy
- Care what you have to say
- Encourage and support you
- Accept you for who you are
- Are happy for you when you do well
- Apologize when they make a mistake
- Give you advice in a caring way
- Keep personal things between the two of you
- Don't pressure you to do things that make you feel uncomfortable

---

About This Chapter: Text under the heading "Friends" is excerpted from "Friendships," girlshealth.gov, Office on Women's Health (OWH), November 2, 2015; Text under the heading "Making New Friends" is excerpted from "Making New Friends," girlshealth.gov, Office on Women's Health (OWH), November 2, 2015; Text under the heading "Dating" is excerpted from "Dating," girlshealth.gov, Office on Women's Health (OWH), November 3, 2015; Text under the heading "Understanding Teen Dating Violence" is excerpted from "Understanding Teen Dating Violence," Centers for Disease Control and Prevention (CDC), 2016.

How Can I Handle Peer Pressure?

Peer pressure is when you do something because friends talk you into it or because you think everyone else is doing it. It can be hard to resist peer pressure. Try to remember that real friends stand by you even if you say "No." Get inspiration and tips for being a great friend and a strong person.

When it's time to stand up for what you believe, be assertive. That means you calmly and politely say what you want (or don't want). You don't need to criticize what the other person is doing. Just keep it simple, like "No, thanks." If you're having trouble handling peer pressure, talk to your parents or a trusted adult. Not sure how to start? You could ask them if they ever had to handle peer pressure when they were young.

How Can I Cope With Cliques?

It's natural to have a group of friends who share things in common. But a clique is a group of friends that is very picky—and even mean—about who can join it. If you are being left out by a clique, try to make friends with people who care about you. It feels good to be liked for who you really are!

How Can I Handle A Fight With A Friend?

You won't always agree with friends. That's natural. But you should always respect each other's thoughts and feelings. Sometimes, a conflict can really hurt or last a long time. How can you cope? Think about whether your friendship is healthy and worth trying to save. If so, you can try some give and take and tips for dealing with conflict.

When Should I End A Friendship?

Sadly, not all friendships last a lifetime. Sometimes friends just grow apart naturally. Sometimes you might need to end a friendship. Signs you should end a friendship include that the person:

- Is mean to you or treats you badly

- Tells your secrets

- Often goes after someone you are dating or like

- Does not want you to have other friends

- Does not listen to you

- Pushes you to do dangerous things

- Blames you for problems in his or her life
- Often tries to control what you do

How Do You End A Relationship?

Sometimes, you can just stop being in touch with your friend. That's a good idea if the person has been emotionally or physically abusive. Other times, a direct talk with the other person is better. That way, your friend won't be confused about what's happening. Also, if you point out the problem, you give the person a chance to change.

Making New Friends

Sometimes, you just feel like branching out and meeting new people. Most of us need different friends for different things. Some friends are great for sharing deep secrets, and others are right for just plain fun. And some are both!

Sometimes, you want new friends because your old friends have been getting in trouble. You can try to help your friends, but it's very important to take care of yourself. If ending the friendship is tough, an adult can offer ideas and support.

It can take practice to figure out how to make new friends. Don't worry if you feel a little shy. The other person may feel exactly the same way and may be very glad you reached out.

You can learn to make new friends. Check out these tips:

1. **Join in!** Get involved in activities that interest you, such as sports, clubs, or volunteering. You'll find people with similar interests.

2. **Say hi.** Introduce yourself to someone new. Repeat the person's name to help you remember it.

3. **Ask questions.** People often love to talk about themselves. Ask where someone got her outfit or what she thinks of the teacher.

4. **Practice.** Are you afraid you'll get tongue-tied? Try out some ideas with an old friend, a sibling, or a parent (or even a patient dog)!

5. **Listen well.** Make eye contact, and avoid distractions like your phone.

6. **Be warm.** Most people appreciate a friendly smile or a kind word.

7. **Be polite.** If someone says something nice to you, make sure to say "thank you."

8. **Suggest something.** Do you have a hard time making conversation? Suggest that you and your new friend do an activity together, like going for a jog or watching a movie.

9. **Be patient.** It can take time to make new friends. Try not to come on too strong by doing things like texting the person many times a day.

10. **Take a risk.** You can't succeed unless you try. Remember, a great new friend may be waiting for you!

Dating

Romance can make your heart pound and your tummy flip. If you're confused or concerned, we can help! Keep reading for answers to common questions about teen dating.

When Do Teens Start Dating?

There is no right age for teens to start dating. Every person is different. Lots of teens enjoy just hanging out in a group. Here are some tips for thinking about when you might start seeing someone:

Ask yourself:

- Do I know what I want in a person I date?

- Is this right for me, or do I just want to do what my friends are doing?

- Am I doing this because I like someone, or because I like the idea of having someone?

- Can I handle tough feelings like jealousy?

- Do I know what I'm ready for in terms of physical stuff?

- Do I know how I'd say no to sex?

Talk to your parents or guardians about starting to date. They may have rules about things like when you can be alone with a date. If you don't like the rules, ask calmly about changing them. Staying calm shows that you're getting more mature. Read about talking with parents.

What Is A Healthy Dating Relationship?

Healthy dating relationships start with the same things that all healthy relationships start with. You can take a quick quiz to help see if your relationship is one to love or one to lose.

You can read some top tips for a healthy dating relationship.

Dating relationships also are different from other relationships. You may have strong feelings of attraction and other intense feelings. You may even want to spend all of your time together. Try to spend some time apart, though. That way you can connect with other people who care about you, too. And you'll have time for goals and activities that matter to you.

What About Dating And Sexual Feelings?

Sexual feelings can be strong, and you may feel confused. Keep in mind that the sex in movies, music, and TV shows often doesn't reflect real or healthy relationships. So how do you know what's right? Trust your instincts and treat yourself with respect—and make sure your crush does, too.

Talk with the other person ahead of time about what you will and will not do physically. Waiting until the heat of the moment to try to cool things down doesn't work as well.

The person you're with should always respect your right to say no.

What about hooking up? Different people mean different things when they say "hooking up." Usually, though, it means doing something sexual with somebody you're not dating. Have you heard that hooking up could be fun? Well, hooking up can have some serious downsides. These include feeling embarrassed or upset afterward, getting pregnant, and getting a sexually transmitted disease (also known as an STI).

Fast Facts About Sex

Do you think most teens are having sex? The truth is 3 out of 4 teens ages 15 to 17 have never had sex.

Do you think sexually transmitted diseases (STDs, or STIs) don't happen to teens? The truth is 1 out of 4 teen girls has an STD.

Should I Date Someone Close To My Age?

It's best to date someone close to your own age. Here are some reasons why:

- Someone older may be more mature and ready for a different kind of relationship.

- Dating someone older increases the odds that your partner will want to have sex before you're ready.

- Younger girls who date older guys are more likely to face an unwanted pregnancy.

- A guy who is legally an adult could get sent to prison if he has sex with you and you're underage. That could happen even if you are 17 and he is 18, depending on the law in your state.

How Can I Stay Safe When Dating?

Dating can be a great way to get to know someone—and to get to know what you want from a relationship. Plus, it can be a lot of fun! But it's not fun to feel scared.

You can take steps to stay safe whenever you go out with someone. For example, try getting to know a person by talking at school or on the phone first. You also can go out with a group of friends to a public place. If the two of you go out alone, tell your parents or guardians who you are going with and where. And follow your parents' rules for things like curfew, since those often are set for your safety. You can read more dating safety tips, including info on sexting.

Understanding Teen Dating Violence

Dating violence is a type of intimate partner violence. It occurs between two people in a close relationship. The nature of dating violence can be physical, emotional, or sexual.

- **Physical**—This occurs when a partner is pinched, hit, shoved, slapped, punched, or kicked.

- **Psychological/Emotional**—This means threatening a partner or harming his or her sense of self-worth. Examples include name calling, shaming, bullying, embarrassing on purpose, or keeping him/her away from friends and family.

- **Sexual**—This is forcing a partner to engage in a sex act when he or she does not or cannot consent. This can be physical or nonphysical, like threatening to spread rumors if a partner refuses to have sex.

- **Stalking**—This refers to a pattern of harassing or threatening tactics that are unwanted and cause fear in the victim.

Dating violence can take place in person or electronically, such as repeated texting or posting sexual pictures of a partner online.

Unhealthy relationships can start early and last a lifetime. Teens often think some behaviors, like teasing and name calling, are a "normal" part of a relationship. However, these behaviors can become abusive and develop into more serious forms of violence.

Why Is Dating Violence A Public Health Problem?

Dating violence is a widespread issue that has serious long-term and short-term effects. Many teens do not report it because they are afraid to tell friends and family.

- Among high school students who dated, 21 percent of females and 10 percent of males experienced physical and/or sexual dating violence.

- Among adult victims of rape, physical violence, and/or stalking by an intimate partner, 22 percent of women and 15 percent of men first experienced some form of partner violence between 11 and 17 years of age.

How Does Dating Violence Affect Health?

Dating violence can have a negative effect on health throughout life. Youth who are victims are more likely to experience symptoms of depression and anxiety, engage in unhealthy behaviors, like using tobacco, drugs, and alcohol, or exhibit antisocial behaviors and think about suicide. Youth who are victims of dating violence in high school are at higher risk for victimization during college.

Who Is At Risk For Dating Violence?

Factors that increase risk for harming a dating partner include the following:

- Belief that dating violence is acceptable

- Depression, anxiety, and other trauma symptoms

- Aggression towards peers and other aggressive behavior

- Substance use

- Early sexual activity and having multiple sexual partners

- Having a friend involved in dating violence

- Conflict with partner

- Witnessing or experiencing violence in the home

Chapter 11

Social Anxiety Disorder: More Than Just Shyness

Are you extremely afraid of being judged by others?

Are you very self-conscious in everyday social situations?

Do you avoid meeting new people?

If you have been feeling this way for at least six months and these feelings make it hard for you to do everyday tasks—such as talking to people at work or school—you may have a social anxiety disorder.

Social anxiety disorder (also called social phobia) is a mental health condition. It is an intense, persistent fear of being watched and judged by others. This fear can affect work, school, and your other day-to-day activities. It can even make it hard to make and keep friends. But social anxiety disorder doesn't have to stop you from reaching your potential. Treatment can help you overcome your symptoms.

What Is Social Anxiety Disorder?

Social anxiety disorder is a common type of anxiety disorder. A person with social anxiety disorder feels symptoms of anxiety or fear in certain or all social situations, such as meeting new people, dating, being on a job interview, answering a question in class, or having to talk to a cashier in a store. Doing everyday things in front of people—such as eating or drinking in front of others or using a public restroom—also causes anxiety or fear. The person is afraid that he or she will be humiliated, judged, and rejected.

About This Chapter: This chapter includes text excerpted from "Social Anxiety Disorder: More Than Just Shyness," National Institute of Mental Health (NIMH), November 2016.

The fear that people with social anxiety disorder have in social situations is so strong that they feel it is beyond their ability to control. As a result, it gets in the way of going to work, attending school, or doing everyday things. People with social anxiety disorder may worry about these and other things for weeks before they happen. Sometimes, they end up staying away from places or events where they think they might have to do something that will embarrass them.

Some people with the disorder do not have anxiety in social situations but have performance anxiety instead. They feel physical symptoms of anxiety in situations such as giving a speech, playing a sports game, or dancing or playing a musical instrument on stage.

Social anxiety disorder usually starts during youth in people who are extremely shy. Social anxiety disorder is not uncommon; research suggests that about 7 percent of Americans are affected. Without treatment, social anxiety disorder can last for many years or a lifetime and prevent a person from reaching his or her full potential.

What Are The Signs And Symptoms Of Social Anxiety Disorder?

When having to perform in front of or be around others, people with social anxiety disorder tend to:

- Blush, sweat, tremble, feel a rapid heart rate, or feel their "mind going blank"

- Feel nauseous or sick to their stomach

- Show a rigid body posture, make little eye contact, or speak with an overly soft voice

- Find it scary and difficult to be with other people, especially those they don't already know, and have a hard time talking to them even though they wish they could

- Be very self-conscious in front of other people and feel embarrassed and awkward

- Be very afraid that other people will judge them

- Stay away from places where there are other people

What Causes Social Anxiety Disorder?

Social anxiety disorder sometimes runs in families, but no one knows for sure why some family members have it while others don't. Researchers have found that several parts of the brain are involved in fear and anxiety. Some researchers think that misreading of others' behavior may play a role in causing or worsening social anxiety. For example, you may think that people are staring or frowning at you when they truly are not. Underdeveloped social skills are another possible contributor to social anxiety. For example, if you have underdeveloped social skills, you may feel discouraged after talking with people and may worry about doing it in the future. By learning more about fear and anxiety in the brain, scientists may be able to create better treatments. Researchers are also looking for ways in which stress and environmental factors may play a role.

How Is Social Anxiety Disorder Treated?

First, talk to your doctor or healthcare professional about your symptoms. Your doctor should do an exam and ask you about your health history to make sure that an unrelated physical problem is not causing your symptoms. Your doctor may refer you to a mental health specialist, such as a psychiatrist, psychologist, clinical social worker, or counselor. The first step to effective treatment is to have a diagnosis made, usually by a mental health specialist.

Social anxiety disorder is generally treated with psychotherapy (sometimes called "talk" therapy), medication, or both. Speak with your doctor or healthcare provider about the best treatment for you. If your healthcare provider cannot provide a referral, visit the National Institute of Mental Health (NIMH) Help for Mental Illnesses webpage at www.nimh.nih.gov/findhelp for resources you may find helpful.

Psychotherapy

A type of psychotherapy called cognitive behavioral therapy (CBT) is especially useful for treating social anxiety disorder. CBT teaches you different ways of thinking, behaving, and reacting to situations that help you feel less anxious and fearful. It can also help you learn and practice social skills. CBT delivered in a group format can be especially helpful.

Support Groups

Many people with social anxiety also find support groups helpful. In a group of people who all have social anxiety disorder, you can receive unbiased, honest feedback about how others in the group see you. This way, you can learn that your thoughts about judgment and rejection are not true or are distorted. You can also learn how others with social anxiety disorder approach and overcome the fear of social situations.

Medication

There are three types of medications used to help treat social anxiety disorder:

- Antianxiety medications

- Antidepressants

- Beta blockers

Antianxiety medications are powerful and begin working right away to reduce anxious feelings; however, these medications are usually not taken for long periods of time. People can build up a tolerance if they are taken over a long period of time and may need higher and higher doses to get the same effect. Some people may even become dependent on them. To avoid these problems, doctors usually prescribe antianxiety medications for short periods, a practice that is especially helpful for older adults.

Antidepressants are mainly used to treat depression, but are also helpful for the symptoms of social anxiety disorder. In contrast to antianxiety medications, they may take several weeks to start working. Antidepressants may also cause side effects, such as headaches, nausea, or difficulty sleeping. These side effects are usually not severe for most people, especially if the dose starts off low and is increased slowly over time. Talk to your doctor about any side effects that you have.

Beta blockers are medicines that can help block some of the physical symptoms of anxiety on the body, such as an increased heart rate, sweating, or tremors. Beta blockers are commonly the medications of choice for the "performance anxiety" type of social anxiety.

Your doctor will work with you to find the best medication, dose, and duration of treatment. Many people with social anxiety disorder obtain the best results with a combination of medication and CBT or other psychotherapies.

Don't give up on treatment too quickly. Both psychotherapy and medication can take some time to work. A healthy lifestyle can also help combat anxiety. Make sure to get enough sleep and exercise, eat a healthy diet, and turn to family and friends who you trust for support.

Finding Help

Mental Health Treatment Program Locator

The Substance Abuse and Mental Health Services Administration (SAMHSA) provides this online resource for locating mental health treatment facilities and programs. The Mental

Health Treatment Locator section of the Behavioral Health Treatment Services Locator lists facilities providing mental health services to persons with mental illness.

Find a facility in your state at www.findtreatment.samhsa.gov.

For additional resources, visit www.nimh.nih.gov/findhelp.

Chapter 12

Bullying And Cyberbullying

What Is Bullying?

Bullying is when a person or a group shows unwanted aggression to another person who is not a sibling or a current dating partner. Cyberbullying (or "electronic aggression") is bullying that is done electronically, including through the Internet, e-mail, or mobile devices, among others.

Bullying can be:

- **Physical**: Punching, beating, kicking, or pushing; stealing, hiding, or damaging another person's belongings; forcing someone to do things against his or her will

- **Verbal**: Teasing, calling names, or insulting another person; threatening another person with physical harm; spreading rumors or untrue statements about another person

- **Relational**: Refusing to talk to someone or making them feel left out; encouraging other individuals to bully someone

To be considered bullying, the behavior in question must be aggressive. The behavior must also involve an imbalance of power (e.g., physical strength, popularity, access to embarrassing details about a person) and be repetitive, meaning that it happens more than once or is highly likely to be repeated.

Bullying also includes cyberbullying and workplace bullying.

About This Chapter: Text beginning with the heading "What Is Bullying?" is excerpted from "Bullying," *Eunice Kennedy Shriver* National Institute of Child Health and Human Development (NICHD), January 28, 2014. Reviewed October 2017; Text beginning with the heading "What Is Cyberbullying?" is excerpted from "Cyberbullying," girlshealth.gov, Office on Women's Health (OWH), April 15, 2014. Reviewed October 2017.

- Cyberbullying has increased with the increased use of the social media sites, the Internet, e-mail, and mobile devices. Unlike more traditional bullying, cyberbullying can be more anonymous and can occur nearly constantly. A person can be cyberbullied day or night, such as when they are checking their e-mail, using Facebook or another social network site, or even when they are using a mobile phone.

- Workplace bullying refers to adult behavior that is repeatedly aggressive and involves the use of power over another person at the workplace. Certain laws apply to adults in the workplace to help prevent such violence.

Who Is Affected And How Many Are At Risk For Bullying?

- A survey from the National Center for Education Statistics (NCES) found that bullying continues to affect many school-aged children: nearly 1 out of 3 students in middle and high school reported that they were bullied at school. Among high school students, 1 out of 9 teens, or about 2.8 million, reported that they had been pushed, shoved, tripped, or spit on during the school year. In the same survey, another 1.5 million high school students reported that they had been threatened with physical harm, and 900,000 had been cyberbullied.

- Data from the Youth Risk Behavior Surveillance System (YRBSS) from the Centers for Disease Control and Prevention (CDC) indicate that about 20 percent of U.S. students in grades 9 through 12 experienced bullying on school property.

- The National Center for Education Statistics (NCES) and Bureau of Justice Statistics (BJS) reported in their School Crime Supplement that about 28 percent of U.S. students in grades 6 through 12 experienced traditional bullying at school. Additionally, during the same school year, 6 percent of students reported being cyberbullied in other places besides at school.

What Are Common Signs Of Being Bullied?

Signs of bullying include:

- Depression, loneliness, or anxiety

- Low self-esteem

- Headaches, stomachaches, tiredness, or poor eating habits

- Missing school, disliking school, or having poorer school performance than previously

- Self-destructive behaviors, such as running away from home or inflicting harm on oneself

- Thinking about suicide or attempting to commit suicide

- Unexplained injuries

- Lost or destroyed clothing, books, electronics, or jewelry

- Difficulty sleeping or frequent nightmares

- Sudden loss of friends or avoidance of social situations

How Does Bullying Affect Health And Well-Being?

Bullying can lead to physical injury, social problems, emotional problems, and even death. Children and adolescents who are bullied are at increased risk for mental health problems, including depression, anxiety, headaches, and problems adjusting to school. Bullying also can cause long-term damage to self-esteem.

Children and adolescents who are bullies are at increased risk for substance use, academic problems, and violence to others later in life.

Children or adolescents who are both bullies and victims suffer the most serious effects of bullying and are at greater risk for mental and behavioral problems than those who are only bullied or who are only bullies.

Eunice Kennedy Shriver National Institute of Child Health and Human Development (NICHD) research studies show that anyone involved with bullying—those who bully others, those who are bullied, and those who bully and are bullied—are at increased risk for depression.

NICHD-funded research studies also found that unlike traditional forms of bullying, youth who are bullied electronically—such as by computer or cell phone—are at higher risk for depression than the youth who bully them. Even more surprising, the same studies found that cyber victims were at higher risk for depression than were cyberbullies or bully-victims (i.e., those who both bully others and are bullied themselves), which was not found in any other form of bullying.

What Are Risk Factors For Being Bullied?

Children who are at risk of being bullied have one or more risk factors:

- Are seen as different from their peers (e.g., overweight, underweight, wear their hair differently, wear different clothing or wear glasses, or come from a different race/ethnicity)

- Are seen as weak or not able to defend themselves

- Are depressed, anxious, or have low self-esteem

- Have few friends or are less popular

- Do not socialize well with others

- Suffer from an intellectual or developmental disability

What Can Be Done To Help Someone Who Is Being Bullied?

Support a child who is being bullied:

- You can listen to the child and let him or her know you are available to talk or even help. A child who is being bullied may struggle talking about it. Consider letting the child know there are other people who can talk with him or her about bullying. In addition, you might consider referring the child to a school counselor, psychologist, or other mental health specialist.

- Give the child advice about what he or she can do. You might want to include role-playing and acting out a bullying incident as you guide the child so that the child knows what to do in a real situation.

- Follow up with the child to show that you are committed to helping put a stop to the bullying.

Address the bullying behavior:

- Make sure a child whom you suspect or know is bullying knows what the problem behavior is and why it is not acceptable.

- Show kids that bullying is taken seriously. If you know someone is being a bully to someone else, tell the bully that bullying will not be tolerated. It is important, however, to demonstrate good behavior when speaking with a bully so that you serve as a role model of good interpersonal behavior.

If you feel that you have taken all possible steps to prevent bullying and nothing has worked, or someone is in immediate danger, there are other ways for you to help.

Table 12.1. Steps To Prevent Bullying

The Problem	What You Can Do
A crime has occurred or someone is at immediate risk of harm.	Call 911.
Someone is feeling hopeless, helpless, or thinking of suicide.	Contact the National Suicide Prevention Lifeline External Web Site Policy online or at 1-800-273-TALK (1-800-273-8255). This toll-free call goes to the nearest crisis center in a national network. These centers provide crisis counseling and mental health referrals.
Someone is acting differently, such as sad or anxious, having trouble completing tasks, or not taking care of themselves.	Find a local counselor or other mental health services.
A child is being bullied in school.	Contact the: • Teacher • School counselor • School coach • School principal • School superintendent • Board of Education
Child is being bullied after school on the playground or in the neighborhood	• Neighborhood watch • Playground security • Team coach • Local precinct/community police
The child's school is not addressing the bullying	Contact the: • School superintendent • Local Board of Education • State Department of Education

What Is Cyberbullying?

Cyberbullying is hurting someone again and again using a computer, a cellphone, or another kind of electronic technology.

Examples of cyberbullying include the following:

- Texting or emailing insults or nasty rumors about someone

- Posting mean comments about someone on Facebook, Twitter, and other social media sites

- Threatening someone through email or other technology

- Tricking someone into sharing embarrassing information

- Forwarding private text messages to hurt or embarrass someone

- Posting embarrassing photos or videos of someone

- Pretending to be someone else online to get that person in trouble or embarrass her

- Creating a website to make fun of someone

How To Prevent Cyberbullying?

Here are some tips that may help protect you from being cyberbullied:

- Don't give out your passwords or personal information. Even your friends could wind up giving your passwords to someone who shouldn't have them.

- Use the privacy options on social networking sites like Facebook, Instagram, and Tumblr that let you choose who can see what you post.

- Don't friend people online if you don't know them, even if you have friends in common.

- Be careful about what you write or what images you send or post because nothing is really private on the Internet.

- If you are using a site like Facebook on a computer in the library, log out before you walk away. If you don't log out, the next person who uses the computer could get into your account.

If You Are Cyberbullied

If you are cyberbullied, you can get help. Here are some important tips:

- If someone bullies you, don't respond. Bullies are looking for a reaction, and you may be able to stop the bullying if you ignore or block the person.

- Save any evidence of cyberbullying, print it out, and show it to a trusted adult.

- Use options that let you block email, cellphone, and text messages from a cyber-bully. You can also stop a person from seeing your Facebook information. If you need help, ask an adult, your cellphone company, or the website where you want to block someone.

- If you are being cyberbullied, ask if your school can get involved.

- Report bullying to your Internet service provider, phone company, email provider, or the website where it happened. Sites like Twitter, YouTube, and Instagram have online forms for reporting.

- Report cyberbullying to police if it involves threats of violence or pornography.

Teen girls say meanness lurks on social media. One out of 5 girls ages 14 to 17 say people of her age are mostly unkind to each other on social media. And one out of 3 girls ages 12 to 13 thought so.

Can you take a second to rewind and be kind before you post?

Some teens think it's easier to get away with bullying online than in person. Also, girls may be more likely to cyberbully than boys. Keep in mind that it's pretty easy to find out who has been cyberbullying. In fact, cyberbullies can get in a lot of trouble with their schools, and possibly even with the police.

Cyberbullying hurts. It can be easier to type something really mean than to say it to a person. But being cyberbullied can sometimes feel even worse than other kinds of bullying. That's because cyberbullying can come at you anytime, anywhere and can reach a lot of people.

Being cyberbullied can make you feel angry, afraid, helpless, and terribly sad. Also, teens who are cyberbullied are more likely than other teens to have problems such as using drugs, skipping school, and even getting sick.

If you are being cyberbullied, talk to an adult you trust. An adult can help you figure out how to handle the problem, and can offer you support.

If you are cyberbullying, it's time to stop. You are not only hurting someone else, you could hurt yourself. You can lose friends and get in trouble with your school or even with the police. If you can't seem to stop yourself from cyberbullying, get help from an adult you trust.

You may hurt someone online without really meaning to do it. It may seem funny to vote for the ugliest kid in school, for example, but try to think about how that person feels. And if you get a message that makes you mad, go away and come back before writing something you may regret. Nearly half of teenage cellphone users say they regretted a text message they sent. Remember, nothing is really secret or private on the Internet, and things you post online can stay there forever.

Sometimes, teens don't want to tell their parents that they are being cyberbullied because they are afraid their parents will take away their phone or computer. If you have this concern, tell your parents, and work with them to figure out a solution. The most important thing is for you to be safe.

Sexting And Cyberbullying

Sexting is sending naked or partly naked photos to someone online or by cellphone. Sometimes, a guy may pressure you to send these kinds of photos. Sometimes, friends may dare you to do it.

It's a very bad idea to send nude photos or forward someone else's. Messages can be traced back to you, and photos can quickly get forwarded to a lot of people. You can really hurt someone's feelings or your own reputation. You can even get in legal trouble for forwarding something that could be considered child pornography.

Examples Of Cyberbullying

Unfortunately, there are lots of ways to hurt someone through technology. Below are some examples.

- **Love, who?**

  Laurie watched as Emma logged on to her account so she could get Emma's password. Later, Laurie logged on as Emma and sent a mean message to Emma's best friend.

- **Picture this!**

  Sue, an overweight high schooler, was changing in the locker room after gym class. Annabelle snapped a pic of Sue with her phone and sent it all around school.

- **Privacy, please!**

  Karen pretended to be Mara's friend and sent her a message asking lots of questions. Mara replied with some really personal info. Karen shared what she said and added her own comment, "Mara is a loser!"

- **Breakup breakdown.**

  After Sarah broke up with Dave, he started texting her constantly at all times of the day and night.

Chapter 13

Sports Pressure And Competition

Negative Outcomes Of Sport Participation

While the research examining the link between sports participation and psychological and social outcomes is predominately positive, not all results have been favorable. For example, research has shown that certain athletes (e.g., those characterized as having high trait anxiety, low perceived competence), when placed in particular situations (e.g., situations where winning is perceived as highly important, event outcomes are very important), experience heightened levels of stress and may even experience burnout and motivational losses.

Factors Influencing Sport Participation And Social And Psychological Outcomes

Two context factors that have been found to influence the beneficial effects of sports participation on social and psychological outcomes are the motivational and caring climates created in the programs. Relative to the motivational climate, the more the climate is task- (focuses on self-improvement) versus ego-involving (focuses on comparison with others), provides autonomy of choice, and enhances enjoyment and positive adult peer relationships, the more likely positive outcomes will result. Overemphasizing winning, employing authoritarian and harsh coaching practices, and engaging in constant social comparison have not been shown to be conducive to the development of social and emotional skills. Creating a caring program climate has also been shown to influence the outcomes of sports participation such as self-efficacy and social behaviors. Specifically, a caring climate is one where "each" participant is

About This Chapter: This chapter includes text excerpted from "Elevate Health—Fitness—Sports—Nutrition," President's Council on Fitness, Sports & Nutrition (PCFSN), 2014. Reviewed October 2017.

treated in a caring and supportive manner. Here, clear expectations relative to the team climate are widely understood by all participants and efforts are made to facilitate positive relationships between all involved.

Role Of Coaches And Sports Parents

The influence of the coach on social and psychological development of the athlete has been the focus of attention for a number of researchers. Results reveal that young athletes who play for coaches who have received training to be more encouraging and supportive in their orientation (versus those who have not) are characterized by a number of positive psychosocial outcomes. These include higher motivation for future involvement, decreased anxiety, increased enjoyment, and enhanced self-esteem. Other studies have shown that young athletes derive more benefits from sports participation if their coaches have philosophies that place importance on the development of socio-emotional life skills in their athletes. More effective coaches also establish trusting relationships with their athletes, intentionally teach life skills and emphasize psychosocial values and skills, spend more time teaching skills like goal setting, help their athletes establish competition strategies, and regularly talk about how sports lessons relate to life.

In addition to coaches, sports parents have been shown to have important influence on their child's youth sports experience. They also serve as role models who provide information about sports involvement, its importance, and how to interact with those in sports. Finally, parents serve as interpreters of their child's sports experience by influencing factors such as perceptions of competence and stress levels. For example, it was found that field hockey players who perceived that their parents placed greater importance on doing well experienced more precompetition cognitive state anxiety than their counterparts who did not perceive such pressure.

Chapter 14

Financial Concerns And Stress

Low Income And Its Effects On Childhood

The negative lifelong effects of adversity and toxic stress in early childhood are well documented. Existing research indicates that children from low-income families face more stressors than children living in advantaged circumstances. Public health research indicates that childhood hardship leads to negative health outcomes and ultimately can impact larger systems such as family units, neighborhoods, and communities. In addition, research suggests that social programs can significantly affect health outcomes and success later in life.

Poverty And Childhood Stress

Childhood poverty is associated with adverse effects on health, educational success, and economic well-being later in life. Hardships associated with persistent poverty leave low-income children more vulnerable to stressors. One of the most prevalent yet preventable types of stressors, material hardships, comes in three forms: food insecurity, unstable or crowded housing, and inability to afford home heating or cooling. As determined by overall measures of wellness, children who experienced multiple poverty-related hardships had significantly

About This Chapter: Text beginning with the heading "Low Income And Its Effects On Childhood" is excerpted from "Insights On Childhood Stress: What Does It Mean For Children In Poverty?" U.S. Department of Housing and Urban Development (HUD), February 9, 2015; Text under the heading "How Teens Can Save And Manage Their Own Money?" is excerpted from "Where To Begin: Saving And Managing Your Own Money," Federal Deposit Insurance Corporation (FDIC), June 10, 2014. Reviewed October 2017; Text under the heading "Managing Real Money In The Real World" is excerpted from "For Teens: How To Ace Your First Test Managing Real Money In The Real World," Federal Deposit Insurance Corporation (FDIC), June 12, 2014. Reviewed October 2017; Text under the heading "How To Cut Down On Spending" is excerpted from "5 Ways To Cut Spending...And Still Get To Do And Buy Cool Things," Federal Deposit Insurance Corporation (FDIC), June 12, 2014. Reviewed October 2017.

worse health outcomes. Severe hardship had a significantly greater impact on health outcomes than moderate hardship, which in turn had a significantly greater impact than no hardship. Investments in home visiting, early education, and public benefit programs could potentially mitigate correctable material hardships.

More than four decades of sociological stress research suggests similar findings regarding the adverse effects of stress and hardship on health. Generational stress, like generational poverty, sustains and widens the health gap between advantaged and disadvantaged social groups. For example, research suggests that stressors proliferate across the life course. Stressful childhood events often generate stressful experiences during young adulthood, leading to more stressors during adulthood. Adults who report multiple traumatic events during childhood report increased recent and lifetime stress levels. Stressors also proliferate across generations. Parental stressors—in particular, the stress of persistent poverty, often manifest in children. Parents under stress give less warmth and support to their children, elevating their children's distress and often leading to behavioral problems and poor educational performance. Systematically, stress proliferation processes are important because they sustain and accelerate social disadvantage across generations.

How Teens Can Save And Manage Their Own Money?

As a teen, you start taking more responsibility for handling money and choosing how you want to save or use it. Here are a few ideas to help make your decisions easier and better.

- **Consider a part-time or summer job.** A job can provide you with additional money as well as new skills, and connections to people who may be helpful after you graduate.

    If you are filling out a job application for a company with a local office, experts say it's generally safe to provide information such as your date of birth and Social Security number (which may be needed for a background check). If you are applying in person, hand the application to the manager (not just any employee), and if you are applying online, make sure you are using the company's legitimate website.

    "But be very suspicious of online job applications for part-time, work-from-home jobs offered by unfamiliar companies without a local office," warned Michael Benardo, Manager of the FDIC's (Federal Deposit Insurance Corporation) Cyber Fraud and Financial Crimes Section. "They may only want to commit identity theft, not hire you."

- **Open a savings account and put money in it for specific goals.** "Some goals will be for the next few weeks or months, while others are for several years away, such as college," said Irma Matias, an FDIC Community Affairs Specialist. Get in the habit of putting at least 10 percent of any gifts or earnings in a savings account right away. Saving a certain percentage of your income before you're tempted to spend it is what financial advisors call "paying yourself first."

  Also think about where you can add to savings by cutting back on spending. "Money you spend today is money you won't have for future wants or needs," added Matias.

- **If you're ready for a checking account, choose one carefully.** Many banks offer accounts geared to teens or other students that require less money to open and charge lower fees than their other accounts. "Even if the account appears to be attractive, think about how you're going to use it—for example, if you mostly want to bank online or with your smartphone—and look into how much that account is likely to cost monthly," said Luke W. Reynolds, Acting Associate Director of the FDIC's Division of Depositor and Consumer Protection (DCP). "Then shop around and compare this account to what is offered by several other institutions."

  When you open an account that comes with a debit card, you will decide how you want the bank to handle an everyday debit card transaction for more than what you have in the account. If you "opt in" (agree) to a bank overdraft program, it will cover these transactions but will charge you a fee of as much as $40 each time. "One overdraft can easily lead to another and become very costly," Reynolds explained. "If you don't opt in, your transactions will be declined, but you won't have to face these penalty fees."

  You may also be able to arrange with your bank to automatically transfer money from a savings account to cover the purchase. You'll probably pay a fee, but it will likely be much less than an overdraft fee.

- **If you're thinking about using a prepaid card instead of a bank account, understand the potential drawbacks.** Prepaid cards often do not offer you the same federal consumer protections as credit or debit cards if, for example, the prepaid card is lost or stolen and used by someone else.

  And, while prepaid cards may advertise no monthly fee, they may charge for making withdrawals, adding money to the card or checking the balance. "It's hard for a prepaid card to beat a well-selected, well-managed checking account for everyday transactions and allowing easy transfers into a savings account," Reynolds concluded.

- **Once you have a bank account, keep a close eye on it.** Watch your balance the best way you can. For example, keep receipts and record expenses so you don't spend more money than you have in your account and run the risk of overdraft costs.

- **Take precautions against identity theft.** Even if you don't have a credit card, you can be targeted by a criminal wanting to use your name to get money or buy goods. So, be very suspicious of requests for your name, Social Security number, passwords, or bank or credit card information.

  "Don't fall for an e-mail, call or text message asking you for financial information," Benardo cautioned. "Never give out any personal information unless you have contacted the company first and you are sure it is legitimate."

- **Understand that borrowing money comes with costs and responsibilities.** When you borrow money, you generally will repay the money monthly and pay interest. Always compare offers to borrow money based on the Annual Percentage Rate (APR). The lower the APR, the less you will pay in interest. And, the longer you take to repay a debt, the more you will pay in interest. If you miss loan payments, you can expect to pay fees and have hard time borrowing money at affordable rates for some time into the future.

Managing Real Money In The Real World

As a teen, you're beginning to make some grown-up decisions about how to save and spend your money. That's why learning the right ways to manage money...right from the start...is important. Here are suggestions.

- **Save some money before you're tempted to spend it.** When you get cash for your birthday or from a job, automatically put a portion of it—at least 10 percent, but possibly more—into a savings or investment account. This strategy is what financial advisors call "paying yourself first." Making this a habit can gradually turn small sums of money into big amounts that can help pay for really important purchases in the future.

  Also put your spare change to use. When you empty your pockets at the end of the day, consider putting some of that loose change into a jar or any other container, and then about once a month put that money into a savings account at the bank.

  "Spare change can add up quickly," said Luke W. Reynolds, Chief of the FDIC's Community Affairs Outreach Section. "But don't let that money sit around your house month after month, earning no interest and at risk of being lost or stolen."

If you need some help sorting and counting your change, he said, find out if your bank has a coin machine you can use for free. If not, the bank may give you coin wrappers.

Some supermarkets and other nonbanking companies have self-service machines that quickly turn coins into cash, but expect to pay a significant fee for the service, often close to 10 cents for every dollar counted, plus you still have to take the cash to the bank to deposit it into your savings account.

- **Keep track of your spending.** A good way to take control of your money is to decide on maximum amounts you aim to spend each week or each month for certain expenses, such as entertainment and snack food. This task is commonly known as "budgeting" your money or developing a "spending plan." And to help manage your money, it's worth keeping a list of your expenses for about a month, so you have a better idea of where your dollars and cents are going.

"If you find you're spending more than you intended, you may need to reduce your spending or increase your income," Reynolds added. "It's all about setting goals for yourself and then making the right choices with your money to help you achieve those goals."

- **Think before you buy.** Many teens make quick and costly decisions to buy the latest clothes or electronics without considering whether they are getting a good value.

"A $200 pair of shoes hawked by a celebrity gets you to the same destination at the same speed as a $50 pair," said Reynolds. "Before you buy something, especially a big purchase, ask yourself if you really need or just want the item, if you've done enough research and comparison-shopping, and if you can truly afford the purchase without having to cut back on spending for something else."

- **Be careful with cards.** Under most state laws, you must be at least 18 years old to obtain your own credit card and be held responsible for repaying the debt. If you're under 18, though, you may be able to qualify for a credit card as long as a parent or other adult agrees to repay your debts if you fail to do so.

An alternative to a credit card is a debit card, which automatically deducts purchases from your savings or checking account. Credit cards and debit cards offer convenience, but they also come with costs and risks that must be taken seriously.

- **Be smart about college.** If you're planning to go to college, learn about your options for saving or borrowing money for what could be a major expense—from tuition to books, fees and housing. Also consider the costs when you search for a school. Otherwise, when you graduate, your college debts could be high and may limit your options when it comes to a career path or where you can afford to live.

How To Cut Down On Spending

Do you want to find ways to stretch your money, so it goes farther and is there when you really need it? Here are some suggestions for knowing how much money you have, how much you need for expenditures, and how to reach your goals by cutting back on what you spend.

1. **Practice self-control.** To avoid making a quick decision to buy something just because you saw it featured on display or on sale:

   - Make a shopping list before you leave home and stick to it.

   - Before you go shopping, set a spending limit (say, $5 or $10) for "impulse buys"— items you didn't plan to buy but that got your attention anyway. If you are tempted to spend more than your limit, wait a few hours or a few days and think it over.

   - Limit the amount of cash you take with you. The less cash you carry, the less you can spend and the less you lose if you misplace your wallet.

2. **Research before you buy.** To be sure you are getting a good value, especially with a big purchase, look into the quality and the reputation of the product or service you're considering. Read "reviews" in magazines or respected website. Talk to knowledgeable people you trust. Check other stores or go online and compare prices. Look at similar items. This is known as "comparison shopping," and it can lead to tremendous savings and better quality purchases. And if you're sure you know what you want, take advantage of store coupons and mail-in "rebates."

3. **Keep track of your spending.** This helps you set and stick to limits, what many people refer to as budgeting. "Maintaining a budget may sound scary or complicated, but it can be as simple as having a notebook and writing down what you buy each month," said Janet Kincaid, FDIC Senior Consumer Affairs Officer. "Any system that helps you know how much you are spending each month is a good thing."

   Also pay attention to small amounts of money you spend. "A snack here and a magazine there can quickly add up," said Paul Horwitz, an FDIC Community Affairs Specialist. He suggested that, for a few weeks, you write down every purchase in a small notebook. "You'll probably be amazed at how much you spend without even thinking."

4. **Think "used" instead of "new."** Borrow things (from the library or friends) that you don't have to own. Pick up used games, DVDs and music at "second-hand" stores around town.

5. **Take good care of what you buy.** It's expensive to replace things. Think about it: Do you really want to buy the same thing twice?

Chapter 15

Violence

Youth Violence[1]

Youth violence is a significant public health problem that affects thousands of young people each day, and in turn, their families, schools, and communities. Youth violence occurs when young people between the ages of 10 and 24 years intentionally use physical force or power to threaten or harm others. Youth violence typically involves young people hurting other peers who are unrelated to them and who they may or may not know well. Youth violence can take different forms. Examples include fights, bullying, threats with weapons, and gang-related violence. A young person can be involved with youth violence as a victim, offender, or witness. Different forms of youth violence can also vary in the harm that results and can include physical harm, such as injuries or death, as well as psychological harm, increased medical and justice costs, decreased property values, and disruption of community services.

Types Of Youth Violence[2]

Youth violence can include:

- Hitting, pinching, punching, or kicking

- Robbery

About This Chapter: This chapter includes text excerpted from documents published by three public domain sources. Text under the heading marked 1 is excerpted from "Youth Violence: Definitions," Centers for Disease Control and Prevention (CDC), June 23, 2017; Text under the headings marked 2 are excerpted from "Violence," girlshealth.gov, Office on Women's Health (OWH), September 16, 2015; Text under the heading marked 3 is excerpted from "Youth Violence: Risk And Protective Factors," Centers for Disease Control and Prevention (CDC), June 23, 2017.

- Using a weapon
- Sexual assault and rape
- Bullying

Individual Risk Factors[3]

Research associates the following risk factors with perpetration of youth violence:

- Poor behavioral control
- Deficits in social cognitive or information-processing abilities
- High emotional distress
- History of treatment for emotional problems
- Antisocial beliefs and attitudes
- Exposure to violence and conflict in the family

What Is A Risk Factor?

A risk factor is a characteristic that increases the likelihood of a person becoming a victim or perpetrator of violence.

(Source: "Preventing Youth Violence: Opportunities For Action," Centers for Disease Control and Prevention (CDC).)

Effects Of Youth Violence[2]

Every year, thousands of young people in the United States die from violence. Violence causes physical injuries, including cuts, bruises, and broken bones. Violence also causes emotional issues, such as being very afraid, nervous, or depressed. Even just seeing violence can lead to serious problems.

Did You Know?

- **Around 2 out of 10** high school girls were in a physical fight in the past year.
- **Nine out of 100** high school girls missed at least one day of school in the past month because they didn't feel safe.

How Can I Stay Away From Violence?[2]

- **Choose your friends carefully.** Stay away from people who are involved in violence. Also try to avoid people who have a hard time controlling how they act when angry.

- **Stick near safe adults.** Hang out where teachers or other responsible adults are around. For after school, consider joining a club, sports, or volunteer activity.

- **Try to stay away from weapons.**

- If a classmate brings a gun, knife, or other weapon to school, tell a teacher or other adult right away.

- If you're out after school and someone is carrying a weapon, leave right away.

- If you have been carrying a weapon to feel safe, talk to an adult about other ways to cope.

- **Learn about safe places.** Try to find out about local places you can go when you feel in danger. These include police stations, firehouses, and libraries. Some places join a special program to help kids in danger. They post a yellow "Safe Place" sign. To find one of these, text your current location to 69866. You can also call 800-786-2929 for help.

- **Practice "safety in numbers."** Try to walk in groups. If you feel in danger while walking alone, go to a place where there are other people as soon as you can.

Are You Involved In Violence?

It is not OK for someone to hurt you, and it is not OK for you to hurt someone else. If you are involved in violence, talk to an adult.

Ways To Help Prevent Violence[2]

- **Lead by example.** Be a model for peace your friends can follow.

- **Speak up.** When people talk about violence, let them know you think it's not OK.

- **Share info.** Suggest ways friends can avoid tough situations: staying away from drugs and alcohol and trying activities that are safe and fun, like sports or a school club.

- **Step in.** If things are getting tense, see if you can help people calm down. If not, don't put yourself in danger. Get the help of an adult.

- **Lend a hand.** Support other people who have been physically or emotionally hurt. That way, you may help them from lashing out as well. Plus, it's just the kind thing to do!

- **Get involved.** See if your school or community has a violence prevention program.

Chapter 16

When Your Parent Has A Substance Abuse Problem

The Relationship Between Substance Use Disorders And Child Maltreatment

It is difficult to provide precise, current statistics on the number of families in child welfare affected by parental substance use or dependency since there is no ongoing, standardized, national data collection on the topic. In a 1999 report to Congress, the U.S. Department of Health and Human Services (HHS) reported that studies showed that between one-third and two-thirds of child maltreatment cases were affected by substance use to some degree. More recent research reviews suggest that the range may be even wider. The variation in estimates may be attributable, in part, to differences in the populations studied and the type of child welfare involvement (e.g., reports, substantiation, out-of-home placement); differences in how substance use (or substance abuse or substance use disorder) is defined and measured; and variations in State and local child welfare policies and practices for case documentation of substance abuse.

Parental Substance Abuse As A Risk Factor For Maltreatment And Child Welfare Involvement

Parental substance abuse is recognized as a risk factor for child maltreatment and child welfare involvement. Research shows that children with parents who abuse alcohol or drugs are more likely to experience abuse or neglect than children in other households. One longitudinal

About This Chapter: This chapter includes text excerpted from "Parental Substance Use And The Child Welfare System," Child Welfare Information Gateway, U.S. Department of Health and Human Services (HHS), October 2014. Reviewed October 2017.

study identified parental substance abuse (specifically, maternal drug use) as one of five key factors that predicted a report to Child Protective Services (CPS) for abuse or neglect. Once a report is substantiated, children of parents with substance use issues are more likely to be placed in out-of-home care and more likely to stay in care longer than other children. The National Survey of Child and Adolescent Well-Being (NSCAW) estimates that 61 percent of infants and 41 percent of older children in out of-home care are from families with active alcohol or drug abuse.

According to data in the Adoption and Foster Care Analysis and Reporting System (AFCARS), parental substance abuse is frequently reported as a reason for removal, particularly in combination with neglect. For almost 31 percent of all children placed in foster care in 2012, parental alcohol or drug use was the documented reason for removal, and in several States that percentage surpassed 60 percent. Nevertheless, many caregivers whose children remain at home after an investigation also have substance abuse issues. NSCAW found that the need for substance abuse services among in-home caregivers receiving child welfare services was substantially higher than that of adults nationwide (29 percent as compared with 20 percent, respectively, for parents ages 18 to 25, and 29 percent versus 7 percent for parents over age 26).

Role Of Co-Occurring Issues

While the link between substance abuse and child maltreatment is well documented, it is not clear how much is a direct causal connection and how much can be attributed to other co-occurring issues. National data reveal that slightly more than one-third of adults with substance use disorders have a co-occurring mental illness. Research on women with substance abuse problems shows high rates of posttraumatic stress disorder (PTSD), most commonly stemming from a history of childhood physical and/ or sexual assault. Many parents with substance abuse problems also experience social isolation, poverty, unstable housing, and domestic violence. These co-occurring issues may contribute to both the substance use and the child maltreatment. Evidence increasingly points to a critical role of stress and reactions within the brain to stress, which can lead to both drug-seeking activity and inappropriate caregiving.

Impact Of Parental Substance Use On Children

The way parents with substance use disorders behave and interact with their children can have a multifaceted impact on the children. The effects can be both indirect (e.g., through a chaotic living environment) and direct (e.g., physical or sexual abuse). Parental substance use can affect parenting, prenatal development, and early childhood and adolescent development.

It is important to recognize, however, that not all children of parents with substance use issues will suffer abuse, neglect, or other negative outcomes.

Parenting

A parent's substance use disorder may affect his or her ability to function effectively in a parental role. Ineffective or inconsistent parenting can be due to the following:

- physical or mental impairments caused by alcohol or other drugs

- reduced capacity to respond to a child's cues and needs

- difficulties regulating emotions and controlling anger and impulsivity

- disruptions in healthy parent-child attachment

- spending limited funds on alcohol and drugs rather than food or other household needs

- spending time seeking out, manufacturing, or using alcohol or other drugs

- incarceration, which can result in inadequate or inappropriate supervision for children

- estrangement from family and other social supports

Family life for children with one or both parents that abuse drugs or alcohol often can be chaotic and unpredictable. Children's basic needs—including nutrition, supervision, and nurturing—may go unmet, which can result in neglect. These families often experience a number of other problems—such as mental illness, domestic violence, unemployment, and housing instability—that also affect parenting and contribute to high levels of stress. A parent with a substance abuse disorder may be unable to regulate stress and other emotions, which can lead to impulsive and reactive behavior that may escalate to physical abuse.

Different substances may have different effects on parenting and safety. For example, the threats to a child of a parent who becomes sedated and inattentive after drinking excessively differ from the threats posed by a parent who exhibits aggressive side effects from methamphetamine use. Dangers may be posed not only from use of illegal drugs, but also, and increasingly, from abuse of prescription drugs (pain relievers, antianxiety medicines, and sleeping pills).

Polysubstance use (multiple drugs) may make it difficult to determine the specific and compounded effects on any individual. Further, risks for the child's safety may differ depending upon the level and severity of parental substance use and associated adverse effects.

Prenatal And Infant Development

The effects of parental substance use disorders on a child can begin before the child is born. Maternal drug and alcohol use during pregnancy have been associated with premature birth, low birth weight, slowed growth, and a variety of physical, emotional, behavioral, and cognitive problems. Research suggests powerful effects of legal drugs, such as tobacco, as well as illegal drugs on prenatal and early childhood development.

Fetal alcohol spectrum disorders (FASD) are a set of conditions that affect an estimated 40,000 infants born each year to mothers who drank alcohol during pregnancy. Children with FASD may experience mild to severe physical, mental, behavioral, and/or learning disabilities, some of which may have lifelong implications (e.g., brain damage, physical defects, and attention deficits). In addition, increasing numbers of newborns—approximately 3 per 1,000 hospital births each year—are affected by neonatal abstinence syndrome (NAS), a group of problems that occur in a newborn who was exposed prenatally to addictive illegal or prescription drugs.

The full impact of prenatal substance exposure depends on a number of factors. These include the frequency, timing, and type of substances used by pregnant women; co-occurring

---

When a woman is pregnant, a baby is growing inside her. If the woman uses drugs while she is pregnant, the drugs can pass to the baby.

Mothers drinking alcohol when pregnant is the most common cause of birth defects that can be avoided.

The baby might:

- be born small
- have problems eating and sleeping
- have problems seeing, hearing, and moving
- be slow to develop

While growing up, the child might:

- have trouble following directions and need to be told things many times
- have trouble paying attention and learning in school
- need special teachers and schools
- have trouble getting along with others
- act out and not understand the effects of doing bad things
- have a drug problem of their own

(Source: "Drug Use Hurts Kids," National Institute on Drug Abuse (NIDA).)

---

environmental deficiencies; and the extent of prenatal care. Research suggests that some of the negative outcomes of prenatal exposure can be improved by supportive home environments and positive parenting practices.

Child And Adolescent Development

Children and youth of parents who use or abuse substances and have parenting difficulties have an increased chance of experiencing a variety of negative outcomes:

- poor cognitive, social, and emotional development

- depression, anxiety, and other trauma and mental health symptoms

- physical and health issues

- substance use problems

Drug Use Hurts Kids

When parents or other family members use drugs, the children can get hurt.

People with drug problems can forget to take care of the kids. There might not be anyone making meals or helping the kids get washed and dressed or dropped off to school. There might not be anyone to buy clothes or do the laundry. There might not be anyone to take the kids to the doctor or help with homework.

Drug use can make parents unable to work and earn money, and make them use up the family's money. The kids might go without heat, food, electricity, or even a place to live.

When family members with drug problems are at home, it may not be safe for the kids. These family members might not be alert enough to protect kids from accidents or from other adults who would harm them. There might be a lot of fighting. They might abuse or neglect the children.

If someone at home is dealing drugs or doing other crimes, it's also dangerous for the kids, and the adults could end up in prison.

(Source: "Drug Use Hurts Kids," National Institute on Drug Abuse (NIDA).)

Parental substance use can affect the well-being of children and youth in complex ways. For example, an infant who receives inconsistent care and nurturing from a parent engaged in addiction-related behaviors may suffer from attachment difficulties that can then interfere with the growing child's emotional development. Adolescent children of parents with substance use disorders, particularly those who have experienced child maltreatment and foster care, may turn to substances themselves as a coping mechanism. In addition, children of parents with substance use issues are more likely to experience trauma and its effects, which include difficulties with concentration and learning, controlling physical and emotional responses to stress, and forming trusting relationships.

Child Welfare Laws Related To Parental Substance Use

In response to concerns over the potential negative impact on children of parental substance abuse and illegal drug-related activities, approximately 47 States and the District of Columbia have child protection laws that address some aspect of parental substance use. Some States have expanded their civil definitions of child abuse and neglect to include a caregiver's use of a controlled substance that impairs the ability to adequately care for a child and/or exposure of a child to illegal drug activity (e.g., sale or distribution of drugs, home-based meth labs). Exposure of children to illegal drug activity is also addressed in 33 States' criminal statutes.

Federal and State laws also address prenatal drug exposure. The Child Abuse Prevention and Treatment Act (CAPTA) requires States receiving CAPTA funds to have policies and procedures for healthcare personnel to notify CPS of substance-exposed newborns and to develop procedures for safe care of affected infants. As yet, there are no national data on CAPTA-related reports for substance-exposed newborns. In some State statutes, substance abuse during pregnancy is considered child abuse and/or grounds for termination of parental rights. State statutes and State and local policies vary widely in their requirements for reporting suspected prenatal drug abuse, testing for drug exposure, CPS response, forced admission to treatment of pregnant women who use drugs, and priority access for pregnant women to State funded treatment programs.

Innovative Prevention And Treatment Approaches

While parental substance abuse continues to be a major challenge in child welfare, the past two decades have witnessed some new and more effective approaches and innovative programs to address child protection for families where substance abuse is an issue. Some examples of promising and innovative prevention and treatment approaches include the following:

- Promotion of protective factors, such as social connections, concrete supports, and parenting knowledge, to support families and buffer risks.

- Early identification of at-risk families in substance abuse treatment programs and through expanded prenatal screening initiatives so that prevention services can be provided to promote child safety and well-being in the home.

- Priority and timely access to substance abuse treatment slots for mothers involved in the child welfare system.

- Gender-sensitive treatment and support services that respond to the specific needs, characteristics, and co-occurring issues of women who have substance use disorders.

- Family-centered treatment services, including inpatient treatment for mothers in facilities where they can have their children with them and programs that provide services to each family member.

- Recovery coaches or mentoring of parents to support treatment, recovery, and parenting.

- Shared family care in which a family experiencing parental substance use and child maltreatment is placed with a host family for support and mentoring.

Chapter 17

Dealing With Divorce

Divorce is the legal breakup of a marriage. Like every major life change, divorce is stressful. It affects finances, living arrangements, household jobs, schedules, and more. If the family includes children, they may be deeply affected.

(Source: "Divorce," National Institutes of Health (NIH).)

The family is the first environment in which youth experience adult relationships. Family composition and adult behaviors—such as the presence of one or both parents and the quality and stability of their relationships—have long-lasting consequences for youth. Past research has consistently shown, for example, that children whose parents divorce are more likely to divorce themselves. Similarly, women born to unmarried mothers are more likely to have a nonmarital birth. Many factors related to family composition, such as income, parenting practices, and stress, could increase the likelihood that teens will have some of the same outcomes as their parents. In addition, the family structure in which children are raised is most familiar, and thus may seem a natural or normal choice when they later form their own families.

About This Chapter: Text in this chapter begins with excerpts from "Pathways To Adulthood And Marriage: Teenagers' Attitudes, Expectations, And Relationship Patterns," U.S. Department of Health and Human Services (HHS), October 2008. Reviewed October 2017; Text under the heading "Impact Of Parental Separation/Divorce" is excerpted from "Pathways To Adulthood And Marriage: Teenagers' Attitudes, Expectations, And Relationship Patterns. What Do Teens Think Of Their Parents' Relationships?" U.S. Department of Health and Human Services (HHS), October 1, 2008. Reviewed October 2017; Text under the heading "What To Do When Parents Divorce?" is excerpted from "Dealing With Loss And Grief," girlshealth.gov, Office on Women's Health (OWH), March 12, 2015; Text under the heading "Overcoming Parents' Divorce" is © 2018 Omnigraphics. Reviewed October 2017.

Impact Of Parental Separation/Divorce

The quality of their parents' relationship has important implications for youth. Past work has shown that parents' marital hostility is associated with behavioral and emotional problems in their children. Some work suggests that it is worse for children for their parents to remain in a conflict-ridden marriage than for their parents to divorce. The parents' relationship may also affect teens' views on marriage and relationships and the quality of their later relationships. For example, a recent study found that adolescent girls with more negative perceptions of the level of conflict in their parents' relationship had greater expectations of unhappiness and divorce in their own future marriages. Similarly, parental conflict after a divorce has been linked with less positive attitudes about marriage among adolescents.

Teens' perceptions of the parental relationship may not be the same as what the parents would say about their own relationship. The teens' perspective, however, is important because it indicates how they are experiencing that relationship. If teens think their parents are always fighting, for example, they are likely to feel stress and turmoil, regardless of whether the parents believe their fighting is frequent. Girls tend to view their parents' relationship more negatively than boys. Girls were more likely to view their parents' marriage as low quality and less likely to perceive the relationship as high quality.

What To Do When Parents Divorce

If your parents are getting divorced, it's normal to feel grief. So much of your life may be changing, and you may not have much control over what happens. You may feel angry, sad, lonely, scared, and lots of other emotions. All this can take time to heal.

There are many things you can do to feel better about a divorce. For starters, you can remember that divorce is never your fault.

Talk to your parents about how you're feeling. Tell them what would make the divorce easier on you. Get help from friends. You might also consider joining a support group for kids of divorcing parents. Your parents, school nurse, school counselor, or other adults can help you look for one. Also, see if you can think about any personal strength that helped you in hard times before.

Overcoming Parents' Divorce

Most teens face anxiety over the future when their parents' divorce. Will they change schools or move to a new house? Will they have to shuttle between parents? Will their financial

Ways To Feel Better

Everybody has the blues sometimes. The good news is that there are things you can do to feel better. Here are some tips to improve your mood:

- **Chill out.** Find a way to relax, such as taking a deep breath or taking a bath.
- **Make a plan.** Life can feel out of control at times. Making a list of what you can do about a problem puts you back in charge.
- **Focus on the positive.** Even in tough times, you likely have some good things going for you.
- **Talk it out.** Talk to your friends, parents or guardians, teachers, counselors, or doctor about what you are feeling. They can help you sort through emotions and find solutions to problems.

(Source: "Feeling Sad," girlshealth.gov, Office on Women's Health (OWH).)

circumstances change? To overcome that fear, teens should discuss their concerns with their parents at the right time when they are most receptive to listening.

Divorce is a life-changing event and causes significant stress for those involved. However, such events also allow individuals to realize their strengths and develop new skills to help them cope. Teens can seek the help of their close relatives, teachers, or counselors to help them in discovering their coping skills. They can find purpose in helping their younger siblings through this shared experience and can, as a result, develop special bonds with them.

Teens can overcome their grief over their parents' divorce by focusing on their own goals and ambitions. By doing so, teens can also reduce their stress and stay on course with their future. They can also take steps to improve their wellbeing by eating properly and exercising regularly. Teens can also distract themselves by concentrating on normal day-to-day activities when they feel depressed or upset.

References

1. Lyness D'Arcy, PhD. "Dealing With Divorce," The Nemours Foundation, January 2015.
2. Lyness D'Arcy, PhD. "Helping Your Child Through A Divorce," The Nemours Foundation, January 2015.

Chapter 18

Family Relationships And Stress

Family Relationships

Many teens have fights or tough times with the adults in their families. They can still have amazing relationships with those adults.

Talking With Parents Or Guardians

As you get older, your relationship with your parents or guardians changes. You may want more privacy or independence, for example. That's natural, but you can still stay connected.

Making time to talk can help strengthen your connections. You might just talk about simple, everyday things or talk while doing something fun together. Being in the habit of talking about small things may make it easier to talk about harder subjects.

If you want to share how you feel about something, it can be easier if you use "I statements." That means you say things like "I feel…" instead of criticizing the other person. Also, if you want something, try to ask politely. (Making demands is not very polite—or very effective.)

If you need to raise a tough topic, keep in mind that your parents or guardians were young once, too. They may have faced very similar issues. Plus, they probably will appreciate your honesty and bravery in coming to them.

If you don't like your family's rules, ask if you can discuss them. Sometimes, parents are willing to change certain rules, especially if you show you can be responsible.

About This Chapter: This chapter includes text excerpted from "Family Relationships: Parents, Stepparents, Grandparents, And Guardians," girlshealth.gov, Office on Women's Health (OWH), November 9, 2015.

Arguing With Parents Or Guardians

Parents and teens disagree and argue at times, even though they love each other.

Tips For Handling Fights With Parents

- **Talk about the rules.** Ask the reasons behind a rule so you can understand it. Consider sharing how a rule makes you feel. Ask if your parents or guardians will consider your ideas about what the rules should be.
- **Follow the rules.** Keep to your curfew if you have one. Call if you're going to be late, so your parents or guardians don't worry. If you follow the rules, your parents or guardians may be more likely to discuss them. If you don't follow the rules, you'll likely just get in trouble.
- **Pick your battles.** Cleaning your room is no fun, but it's most likely not worth fighting about.
- **Spend time with your family.** Some teens fight with their parents or guardians over how much time they spend with friends. Talk it over, and make some special family time. You might go for a walk or have dinner together.
- **Try to stay calm.** Don't yell or stomp your feet when your parents or guardians say no. If you listen and speak calmly, you may show them that you are growing up.
- **After an argument, think about what happened.** Consider your part in the problem, and apologize. Talk about how you might prevent similar fights in the future.

Handling Challenging Times

Lots of teens face some really scary family issues, like illness and divorce. Over time, they usually feel better. Here are some ways you can feel better, too. Think of ways you can cope, like going for a walk, doing something creative, or talking to a friend. Stay away from things like drugs and drinking, since they only make problems worse.

If you need support from outside your family, talk to a trusted adult, such as a teacher, religious leader, or school counselor. You also can contact a 24-hour crisis text line and a helpline for kids and teens.

Keep reading for information on coping in some specific situations.

- Do you take care of someone in your family?

- Are you struggling because your parents are getting divorced? Remember, divorce is never a kid's fault. With time and support, you can adjust to the changes you're facing.

- Does your parent or other relative have an illness or disability?

- Do you have a relative in the military?

- Is your family having money problems?

- Does your parent have a drug or alcohol problem?

Few things in life are harder than the death of a close relative.

Getting Along With Stepparents

A new stepparent can bring up lots of feelings. Even if you like your stepparent, you may feel sad, worried, or upset at times.

Here are some tips that can help:

- **Accept your feelings.** It's natural to have feelings like confusion, anger, and guilt when a parent remarries. Don't worry that there's something wrong with you if you have any (or all) of these feelings!

- **Sort through your feelings.** Keeping a journal might help. Friends who have gone through a similar situation may also be able to offer tips.

- **Talk honestly.** If you don't like any new rules or situations, ask calmly and respectfully about changing them. Check out tips for handling conflict.

- **Get support from your parent or another trusted adult.** Adults who care about you really want to help. If it seems too hard to turn to a family member, talk to another adult you trust. If you are struggling, a mental health professional like a school counselor can help.

- **Try to spend time with your stepparent.** This new person is going to be around, and chances are you will be happier if you can find his or her more positive sides.

Keep in mind that with patience—and some hard work—lots of stepfamilies end up feeling very close.

Chapter 19

Moving

Moving away from home can be overwhelming for many people. For most teens it is frightening and exciting at the same time. Moving is a major decision that requires a lot of planning, discussion, and action. The decision to relocate might cause distress, and the experience could be traumatic for some individuals. Whatever the reason for the move, it is important to prepare well and take care of yourself to make the change less stressful. You should consider all the relevant factors, make detailed plans, and have a strategy in place to make the change as easy as possible.

Reasons To Move From Home

There can be numerous reasons for moving. Teens leave home for college, or parents may be transferred resulting in the entire family moving to another city, state, or even overseas. Some people move because they wish to live independently or do not get along with their parents, while others are forced to move to escape abuse and violence at home. Here's a look at a few of these reasons in more detail:

- **Relocating with family.** It can be very difficult to come to terms with decision to move an entire family. You cannot expect to be uprooted and feel right at home in a new place immediately. When a family is in the process of moving, parents can be busy with all the details and not realize how the change is affecting their children. If you can't deal with feelings of sadness or anxiety, talk to your parents or another adult who will be helpful and supportive. Although most people begin feeling better once they've settled down after moving, if you suppress your feelings, you could end up with problems later. Even

About This Chapter: "Moving," © 2018 Omnigraphics. Reviewed October 2017.

though moving is stressful, the impact it causes can be eased. For example, although children may find it difficult to say goodbye to friends, it is easy these days to stay in touch by phone and social media, sharing pictures and videos. Children may also have to give up sports training or ballet and other activities, which could create additional anxiety. Teens can research the Internet and learn about life and culture in their new community. They can locate places of interest, sports clubs, and training facilities where they can continue with practice and engage in their usual activities. As newcomers to a community, children will also have to get accustomed to new societal customs, some of which can be found online. A change of school will also likely be on the cards. The way things are done in the new school might vary, and text books could be different. You may not be on the same level academically as your peers in the new school, depending on the previous curriculum you were in. Teachers will always be ready to help you out once they know you've relocated. Children who are not very good in academics or have had difficulty with peers might feel excited at the prospect of making a fresh beginning and new friends, although it's best not to have unreasonable expectations in this regard. You carry along your personal strengths, weaknesses, likes, and dislikes when you move. On the other hand, there are many new opportunities that await young people when they move. They have the opportunity to live in a new city, learn its culture and traditions, and meet new friends.

- **Leaving home for college.** Many teens experience living independently for the first time when they begin their college education. Going to college means leaving familiar territory behind. This could be a dream come true or a nightmare, depending on the situation and personal viewpoint. Whatever the case, leaving home could be stressful, and it's easy to ignore signs of stress when you're caught up in the hectic moving process. Students are usually informed about their future roommates a few weeks before relocating to college. It's easy to contact people over social networks these days, have a discussion, make plans, and build aback rapport with your roommate. This way you can feel comfortable when you move into the dorm and meet your roommate in person for the first time. If you talk in advance, you can decide about sharing things, what each of you will bring, and discuss bunk arrangements. The act of moving itself may be stressful. You will need to make a list and decide what to take along and what leave behind. Pack items you know you're going to use for sure and leave the rest. You can always get it later, have it shipped to you, or buy it on campus. If you pack too much, it might become difficult to share dorm space with your roommate. Students starting college face an incredible amount of stress, and the transition is not always easy. Check with your school to know whom to contact for support and emergency services, such as counseling, hospitals, police, and firefighters. It's possible you won't need these services, but if you do, it's good to be prepared. And don't hesitate to seek help from your family and friends. Having people assist you will get you moved into your room without getting exhausted. Try to develop coping skills to help you deal with stress. For example, continuing to enjoy familiar hobbies and activities can help you ease into college life and keep you engaged. Singing, drawing, video games, walking, biking, and exercise are some things you can do, both for fun and to help you feel better when you are upset.

- **Leaving home to live independently.** When you think it's time for you to lead an independent life, you could begin thinking about leaving home. It's wise to consult someone you trust before making the final decision, but in the end the choice is yours, and you should clearly understand what is involved and what the consequences will be. Talking to another person will help you gain a good perspective on what to expect, clarify your future goals, and plan for how to achieve them. Staying at home is usually cheaper, more conducive to study, and often comes with a built-in support system. Take into account how you will manage your emotional, physical, and financial needs if you live independently. Make sure you've made a realistic analysis of what to expect. There are numerous factors to consider when looking for a place to live. Of primary consideration is choosing something that is within your budget. Location is another important factor, since you may need to be close to public transportation facilities, as well as other utilities and services. If you are working, then you'll need to plan a detailed budget for food, rent, utilities, and transportation.

- **Leaving home because of conflict.** Do not make a rash decision about moving in the middle of a conflict. Don't storm out because of a fight without first trying your best to resolve the issues at home. Consider all the factors carefully before moving out. Be sure you're leaving for the right reasons and not just making an impulsive, emotional decision. One critical consideration is ensuring that you will be able to support yourself financially if you decide to live on your own. If you're leaving home because of conflict, abuse, or violence, it is possible that you may have a hard time finding safe accommodations very quickly. If you're young and cannot cope with living alone, seek help from community organizations and government agencies. It could be difficult if you are leaving in a hurry, but remember that your personal safety is paramount. Enlist the help of an adult, family member, or friend to locate a safe place to stay. Contact the local police or call emergency services if you think you are in danger. When people leave home because of conflict, abuse, or violence, it may be easy to make the decision move out, but it is not the only choice. Consider resolving issues with parents and other family members by communicating and dealing with all the individuals involved. You could benefit from the services of a professional counselor to help gain fresh perspective on the situation.

Handling Relationship Concerns

Living independently and establishing your own life is a normal part of growing up, but it can be challenging for parents to come to terms with it, since they've been involved in your life and decisions for so long. They could feel rejected and sad when you leave home, so keep in mind that this is a huge transition for your parents, as well. They'll feel better if you include them in your planning process, let them know you appreciate them, and assure them that they'll still be an important part of your life.

Siblings, too, can have a hard time when a teen leaves for college. Younger brothers and sisters may feel the same sense of loss that parents experience, and these feelings can become overwhelming for them. Young siblings frequently look up to their older brothers and sisters, relying on them for guidance and advice, and they may become apprehensive at the thought of losing that support. You can help by involving them in the moving process and making a special effort to stay in touch after you relocate.

The Positive Aspects Of Moving

Moving is a difficult choice, but you will almost certainly find that you have gained some valuable skills in the process. You'll learn that you know how to make new friends, be flexible, and find your way in new places. Even though it may have been tough for you in the beginning, you might discover that you actually like the new place even better.

References

1. "College Move-In Stress: How To Reduce It," Teen Lifeline, June 29, 2016.

2. "Helping Children Adjust To A Move," American Academy of Pediatrics, June 1, 2007.

3. Lyness, D'Arcy, PhD. "The Moving Blues," The Nemours Foundation, October 2013.

4. "Moving Out Of Home—Tips For Young People," State of Victoria, June, 2016.

5. Powell-Lunder, Jennifer, Psy.D. "College Bound: The Impact On The Siblings Left Behind," Huffington Post, October 8, 2013.

Part Three
Effects Of Stress On The Body, Mind, And Behavior

Chapter 20

The Stress Response And How It Can Affect You

The stress response, or "fight or flight" response is the emergency reaction system of the body. It is there to keep you safe in emergencies. The stress response includes physical and

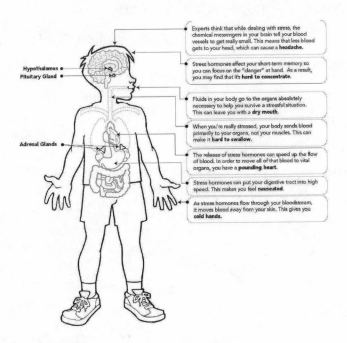

Hypothalamus
Pituitary Gland

Adrenal Glands

Experts think that while dealing with stress, the chemical messengers in your brain tell your blood vessels to get really small. This means that less blood gets to your head, which can cause a **headache**.

Stress hormones affect your short-term memory so you can focus on the "danger" at hand. As a result, you may find that it's **hard to concentrate**.

Fluids in your body go to the organs absolutely necessary to help you survive a stressful situation. This can leave you with a **dry mouth**.

When you're really stressed, your body sends blood primarily to your organs, not your muscles. This can make it **hard to swallow**.

The release of stress hormones can speed up the flow of blood. In order to move all of that blood to vital organs, you have a **pounding heart**.

Stress hormones can put your digestive tract into high speed. This makes you feel **nauseated**.

As stress hormones flow through your bloodstream, it moves blood away from your skin. This gives you **cold hands**.

Figure 20.1. Stress Response

(Source: "The Body-Mind Connection Of Stress," Centers for Diseases Control and Prevention (CDC).)

About This Chapter: This chapter includes text excerpted from "The Stress Response And How It Can Affect You," U.S. Department of Veterans Affairs (VA), July 2013. Reviewed October 2017.

thought responses to your perception of various situations. When the stress response is turned on, your body may release substances like adrenaline and cortisol.

Your organs are programmed to respond in certain ways to situations that are viewed as challenging or threatening. The stress response can work against you. You can turn it on when you don't really need it and, as a result, perceive something as an emergency when it's really not. It can turn on when you are just thinking about past or future events. Harmless, chronic conditions can be intensified by the stress response activating too often, with too much intensity, or for too long.

Stress responses can be different for different individuals. Below is a list of some common stress responses can be different for different individuals. Below is a list of some common stress related responses people have.

Physical Responses

- Muscle aches
- Heart rate
- Weight gain
- Constipation
- Muscle twitching
- Low energy
- Tight chest
- Dizziness
- Stomach
- Cramps
- Insomnia
- Headache
- Nausea
- Dry mouth
- Weight loss
- Weakness

- Diarrhea
- Trembling
- Chills
- Sweating
- Choking feeling
- Leg cramps
- Hot flashes
- Pounding
- Heart
- Chest pain
- Numb or
- Tingling
- Hands/Feet
- Blood Pressure
- Dry throat
- Face flushing

- Feeling faint
- Neck pain

- Urination
- Lightheadedness

Emotional And Thought Responses

- Restlessness
- Agitation
- Worthlessness
- Depression
- Guilt
- Anger
- Nightmares
- Sensitivity
- Numbness
- Mood swings
- Concentration
- Preoccupation

- Insecurity
- Anxiety
- Depression
- Hopelessness
- Defensiveness
- Racing thoughts
- Intense thinking
- Expecting the worst
- Lack of motivation
- Forgetfulness
- Rigidity
- Intolerance

Behavioral Responses

- Avoidance
- Neglect
- Smoking
- Poor appearance
- Spending
- Eating
- Nail biting
- Talking
- Sexual problems

- Fidgeting
- Exercise
- Aggressive speaking
- Sleeping
- Relaxing activities
- Withdrawal
- Alcohol use
- Eating
- Arguing

- Poor Hygiene
- Seeking reassurance
- Skin picking
- Body checking
- Foot tapping

- Rapid walking
- Teeth clenching
- Multitasking
- Fun activities

The parasympathetic nervous system in your body is designed to turn on your body's relaxation response. Your behaviors and thinking can keep your body's natural relaxation response from operating at its best.

Getting your body to relax on a daily basis for at least brief periods can help decrease unpleasant stress responses. Learning to relax your body, through specific breathing and relaxation exercises as well as by minimizing stressful thinking, can help your body's natural relaxation system be more effective. Your behavioral healthcare provider can assist you with learning relaxation techniques.

Chapter 21

Effects Of Childhood Stress On Health Across The Lifespan

Stress is an inevitable part of life. Human beings experience stress early, even before they are born. A certain amount of stress is normal and necessary for survival. Stress helps children develop the skills they need to cope with and adapt to new and potentially threatening situations throughout life. Support from parents and/or other concerned caregivers is necessary for children to learn how to respond to stress in a physically and emotionally healthy manner.

> Stress is internal or external influences that disrupt an individual's normal state of well-being. These influences are capable of affecting health by causing emotional distress and leading to a variety of physiological changes. These changes include increased heart rate, elevated blood pressure, and a dramatic rise in hormone levels.

The beneficial aspects of stress diminish when it is severe enough to overwhelm a child's ability to cope effectively. Intensive and prolonged stress can lead to a variety of short- and long-term negative health effects. It can disrupt early brain development and compromise functioning of the nervous and immune systems. In addition, childhood stress can lead to health problems later in life including alcoholism, depression, eating disorders, heart disease, cancer, and other chronic diseases.

The purpose of this chapter is to summarize the research on childhood stress and its implications for adult health and well-being. Of particular interest is the stress caused by child abuse, neglect, and repeated exposure to intimate partner violence (IPV).

About This Chapter: This chapter includes text excerpted from "The Effects Of Childhood Stress On Health Across The Lifespan," Centers for Disease Control and Prevention (CDC), 2008. Reviewed October 2017.

Types Of Stress

Following are descriptions of the three types of stress that The National Scientific Council on the Developing Child (NSCDC) has identified based on available research:

Positive stress results from adverse experiences that are short-lived. Children may encounter positive stress when they attend a new daycare, get a shot, meet new people, or have a toy taken away from them. This type of stress causes minor physiological changes including an increase in heart rate and changes in hormone levels. With the support of caring adults, children can learn how to manage and overcome positive stress. This type of stress is considered normal and coping with it is an important part of the development process.

Tolerable stress refers to adverse experiences that are more intense but still relatively short-lived. Examples include the death of a loved one, a natural disaster, a frightening accident, and family disruptions such as separation or divorce. If a child has the support of a caring adult, tolerable stress can usually be overcome. In many cases, tolerable stress can become positive stress and benefit the child developmentally. However, if the child lacks adequate support, tolerable stress can become toxic and lead to long-term negative health effects.

Toxic stress results from intense adverse experiences that may be sustained over a long period of time—weeks, months or even years. An example of toxic stress is child maltreatment, which includes abuse and neglect. Children are unable to effectively manage this type of stress by themselves. As a result, the stress response system gets activated for a prolonged amount of time. This can lead to permanent changes in the development of the brain. The negative effects of toxic stress can be lessened with the support of caring adults. Appropriate support and intervention can help in returning the stress response system back to its normal baseline.

The Effects Of Toxic Stress On Brain Development In Early Childhood

The ability to manage stress is controlled by brain circuits and hormone systems that are activated early in life. When a child feels threatened, hormones are released and they circulate throughout the body. Prolonged exposure to stress hormones can impact the brain and impair functioning in a variety of ways.

- Toxic stress can impair the connection of brain circuits and, in the extreme, result in the development of a smaller brain.

- Brain circuits are especially vulnerable as they are developing during early childhood. Toxic stress can disrupt the development of these circuits. This can cause an individual to develop a low threshold for stress, thereby becoming overly reactive to adverse experiences throughout life.

- High levels of stress hormones, including cortisol, can suppress the body's immune response. This can leave an individual vulnerable to a variety of infections and chronic health problems.

- Sustained high levels of cortisol can damage the hippocampus, an area of the brain responsible for learning and memory. These cognitive deficits can continue into adulthood.

The Effects Of Toxic Stress On Adult Health And Well-Being

Research findings demonstrate that childhood stress can impact adult health. The adverse childhood experiences (ACE) study is particularly noteworthy because it demonstrates a link between specific

1. Violence–related stressors, including child abuse, neglect, and repeated exposure to intimate partner violence, and

2. Risky behaviors and health problems in adulthood.

The Adverse Childhood Experiences (ACEs) Study

The ACE Study, a collaboration between the Centers for Disease Control and Prevention (CDC) and Kaiser Permanente's Health Appraisal Clinic in San Diego, uses a retrospective approach to examine the link between childhood stressors and adult health. Over 17,000 adults participated in the research, making it one of the largest studies of its kind. Each participant completed a questionnaire that asked for detailed information on their past history of abuse, neglect, and family dysfunction as well as their current behaviors and health status. Researchers were particularly interested in participants' exposure to the following ten ACEs:

- Abuse

- Emotional

- Physical

- Sexual

- Neglect

- Emotional

- Physical

- Household dysfunction

- Mother treated violently

- Household substance abuse

- Household mental illness

- Parental separation or divorce

- Incarcerated household member

Chapter 22

Adverse Childhood Experiences (ACEs)

Understanding Adverse Childhood Experiences (ACEs)[1]

Adverse childhood experiences (ACEs) are a significant risk factor for substance use disorders and can impact prevention efforts. They are stressful or traumatic events, including abuse and neglect. They may also include household dysfunction such as witnessing domestic violence or growing up with family members who have substance use disorders. ACEs are strongly related to the development and prevalence of a wide range of health problems throughout a person's lifespan, including those associated with substance misuse.

ACEs include:

- Physical abuse

- Sexual abuse

- Emotional abuse

- Physical neglect

- Emotional neglect

- Intimate partner violence

About This Chapter: This chapter includes text excerpted from documents published by two public domain sources. Text under the headings marked 1 are excerpted from "Adverse Childhood Experiences," Substance Abuse and Mental Health Services Administration (SAMHSA), September 5, 2017; Text under heading marked 2 is excerpted from "Child Abuse And Neglect: Consequences," Centers for Disease Control and Prevention (CDC), March 28, 2016.

- Mother treated violently

- Substance misuse within household

- Household mental illness

- Parental separation or divorce

- Incarcerated household member

ACEs are a good example of the types of complex issues that the prevention workforce often faces. The negative effects of ACEs are felt throughout the nation and can affect people of all backgrounds. Successfully addressing their impact requires:

- Assessing prevention needs and gathering data

- Effective and sustainable prevention approaches guided by applying the Strategic Prevention Framework (SPF)

- Prevention efforts aligned with the widespread occurrence of ACEs

- Building relationships with appropriate community partners through strong collaboration

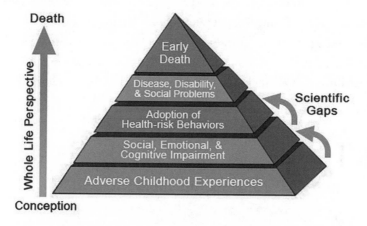

Figure 22.1. Adverse Childhood Experiences Pyramid

Child Abuse And Neglect: Consequences[2]

Child abuse and neglect affect children's health now and later, and costs to our country are significant. Neglect, physical abuse, custodial interference, and sexual abuse are types of child maltreatment that can lead to poor physical and mental health well into adulthood.

The physical, psychological, behavioral and economic consequences of child maltreatment are explained below.

> ## Prevalence: 1 In 4 Children Suffer Abuse
>
> An estimated 702,000 children were confirmed by child protective services as being victims of abuse and neglect in 2014. At least one in four children have experienced child neglect or abuse (including physical, emotional, and sexual) at some point in their lives, and one in seven children experienced abuse or neglect in the last year.

Effects: Child Abuse And Neglect Affect Children Now And Later

- Improper brain development

- Impaired cognitive (learning ability) and socio-emotional (social and emotional) skills

- Lower language development

- Blindness, cerebral palsy from head trauma

- Higher risk for heart, lung and liver diseases, obesity, cancer, high blood pressure, and high cholesterol

- Anxiety

- Smoking, alcoholism, and drug abuse

Physical

- In 2014, approximately 1,580 children died from abuse and neglect across the country—a rate of 2.13 deaths per 100,000 children.

- Abuse and neglect during infancy or early childhood can cause regions of the brain to form and function improperly with long-term consequences on cognitive and language abilities, socioemotional development, and mental health. For example, the stress of chronic abuse may cause a "hyperarousal" response in certain areas of the brain, which may result in hyperactivity and sleep disturbances.

- Children may experience severe or fatal head trauma as a result of abuse. Nonfatal consequences of abusive head trauma include varying degrees of visual impairment (e.g., blindness), motor impairment (e.g., cerebral palsy) and cognitive impairments.

- Children who experience abuse and neglect are also at increased risk for adverse health effects and certain chronic diseases as adults, including heart disease, cancer, chronic lung disease, liver disease, obesity, high blood pressure, high cholesterol, and high levels of C-reactive protein.

Psychological

- In one long-term study, as many as 80 percent of young adults who had been abused met the diagnostic criteria for at least one psychiatric disorder at age 21. These young adults exhibited many problems, including depression, anxiety, eating disorders, and suicide attempts.

- The stress of chronic abuse may result in anxiety and may make victims more vulnerable to problems, such as posttraumatic stress disorder, conduct disorder, and learning, attention, and memory difficulties.

Behavioral

- Children who experience abuse and neglect are at increased risk for smoking, alcoholism, and drug abuse as adults, as well as engaging in high-risk sexual behaviors.

- Those with a history of child abuse and neglect are 1.5 times more likely to use illicit drugs, especially marijuana, in middle adulthood.

- Studies have found abused and neglected children to be at least 25 percent more likely to experience problems such as delinquency, teen pregnancy, and low academic achievement. Similarly, a longitudinal study found that physically abused children were at greater risk of being arrested as juveniles, being a teen parent, and less likely to graduate high school.

- A National Institute of Justice study indicated that being abused or neglected as a child increased the likelihood of arrest as a juvenile by 59 percent. Abuse and neglect also increased the likelihood of adult criminal behavior by 28 percent and violent crime by 30 percent.

- Child abuse and neglect can have a negative effect on the ability of both men and women to establish and maintain healthy intimate relationships in adulthood.

ACEs And Prevention Efforts[1]

Preventing ACEs and engaging in early identification of people who have experienced them could have a significant impact on a range of critical health problems.

You can strengthen your substance misuse prevention efforts by:

- Informing local decision-making by collecting state- and county-level ACEs data

- Increasing awareness of ACEs among state- and community-level substance misuse prevention professionals, emphasizing the relevance of ACEs to behavioral health disciplines

- Including ACEs among the primary risk and protective factors when engaging in prevention planning efforts

- Selecting and implementing programs, policies, and strategies designed to address ACEs, including efforts focusing on reducing intergenerational transmission of ACEs

- Using ACEs research and local ACEs data to identify groups of people who may be at higher risk for substance use disorders and to conduct targeted prevention

Chapter 23

Stress And Your Immune System

Everyone feels stressed from time to time. Stress can give you a rush of energy when it's needed most—for instance, competing in sports, working on an important project, or facing a dangerous situation. The hormones and other chemicals released when under stress prepare you for action. You breathe faster, your heartbeat quickens, blood sugar rises to give you energy, and your brain uses more oxygen as it shifts into high alert.

Your Immune System

The immune system protects the body from infections and diseases. It's sometimes also called the lymphatic system. It's made up of the tissues and organs that produce, store, and carry white blood cells that fight infections and other diseases. This system includes the bone marrow, spleen, tonsils, thymus, lymph nodes, and lymphatic vessels.

(Source: "BAM! Body And Mind—Your Immune System," Centers for Disease Control and Prevention (CDC).)

But if stress lasts a long time—a condition known as chronic stress—those "high-alert" changes become harmful rather than helpful. "Stress clearly promotes higher levels of inflammation, which is thought to contribute too many diseases of aging. Inflammation has been linked to cardiovascular disease, diabetes, arthritis, frailty, and functional decline," says Dr.

About This Chapter: Text in this chapter begins with excerpts from "Feeling Stressed?—Stress Relief Might Help Your Health," *NIH News in Health*, National Institutes of Health (NIH), December 2014. Reviewed October 2017; Text beginning with the heading "Chronic Stress And Immune Dysregulation" is excerpted from "Kiecolt-Glaser Offers New Paradigm On How Stress Kills," National Institutes of Health (NIH), August 8, 2008. Reviewed October 2017.

Janice Kiecolt-Glaser, a leading stress researcher at Ohio State University (OSU). She and other researchers have found that stress affects the body's immune system, which then weakens your response to vaccines and impairs wound healing. Research has linked chronic stress to digestive disorders, urinary problems, headaches, sleep difficulties, depression, and anxiety.

Chronic Stress And Immune Dysregulation

The idea that the mind affects health and illness is thousands of years old, but only in recent decades have scientists tracked down the data.

How do scientists prove the effects of stress on health? One path is to follow the cytokines, among the most crucial proteins in the body. Cytokines, including the interleukins, carry messages vital to immune response. Part of that response is inflammation. As one of the body's normal defenses against infection, injury, irritation or surgery, inflammation is not the same as infection. And acute inflammation is not the same as chronic.

"We need good inflammation," said Kiecolt-Glaser, "because cytokines attract immune cells. With acute inflammation, good things happen. With chronic inflammation, you have troubles, because of its association with tumor cell survival" and other harms.

It's an intricate process. Imagine tumbling down a ladder in a cascade of negative effects:

- Chronic stress can cause immune dysregulation.

- This dysregulation causes increased risk of disease.

- And that risk in turn increases the proinflammatory cytokines, including interleukin-6 (IL-6).

Some highlights on how chronic stress affects health:

- Chronic stress substantially accelerates age-related changes in IL-6, a cytokine linked to some cancers, cardiovascular disease, type II diabetes, osteoporosis, arthritis, frailty and function decline. "It's a new paradigm," Kiecolt-Glaser said. "Cholesterol and the immune system work together to cause heart disease and stroke."

- When dental students on vacation were compared to those taking "a particularly dreaded exam—immunology," no student healed as rapidly during exams. Oral wound-healing took them 40 percent longer.

- Personal relationships influence immune/endocrine function and health. Hostile couples' wounds healed more slowly after conflict.

- Women show larger response to interpersonal stress.

The Good Guys

The players in the immune system include:

- **Lymph**—A clear fluid that travels through the lymphatic system and carries cells that help fight infections and other diseases.

- **Lymph nodes**—Rounded masses of lymphatic tissue that is surrounded by a capsule of connective tissue. Lymph nodes filter lymph, and they store white blood cells. They are located along lymphatic vessels.

- **Lymph vessels**—Thin tubes that carry lymph and white blood cells through the lymphatic system. They branch, like blood vessels, into all the tissues of the body.

- **The thymus**—An organ in the chest behind the breastbone. T lymphocytes grow and multiply in the thymus.

- **The spleen**—An organ on the left side of the abdomen, near the stomach. It produces some white blood cells, filters the blood, stores blood cells, and destroys old blood cells.

- **White blood cells**—Cells are made by bone marrow and help the body fight infection and other diseases. There are lots of types of white blood cells.

The Enemy

- **Antigen**—A foreign substance that causes a response in the immune system. Antigens can be bacterium, viruses, etc. There's a different antigen for every cold that you've ever had and every type of flower that's ever made you sneeze.

How It Works

White blood cells patrol the body. When they come across an antigen, they produce an antibody. The antibody binds to the antigen. Each antigen is shaped differently. The immune system has to produce the antibody that fits it exactly. Some antibodies destroy antigens when they bind with them. Others make it easier for white blood cells to destroy the antigen.

(Source: "BAM! Body And Mind—Your Immune System," Centers for Disease Control and Prevention (CDC).)

Chapter 24

Stress And Cancer

What Is Psychological Stress?

Psychological stress describes what people feel when they are under mental, physical, or emotional pressure. Although it is normal to experience some psychological stress from time to time, people who experience high levels of psychological stress or who experience it repeatedly over a long period of time may develop health problems (mental and/or physical).

Stress can be caused both by daily responsibilities and routine events, as well as by more unusual events, such as a trauma or illness in oneself or a close family member. When people feel that they are unable to manage or control changes caused by cancer or normal life activities, they are in distress. Distress has become increasingly recognized as a factor that can reduce the quality of life of cancer patients. There is even some evidence that extreme distress is associated with poorer clinical outcomes. Clinical guidelines are available to help doctors and nurses assess levels of distress and help patients manage it.

This chapter provides a general introduction to the stress that people may experience as they cope with cancer.

How Does The Body Respond During Stress?

The body responds to physical, mental, or emotional pressure by releasing stress hormones (such as epinephrine and norepinephrine) that increase blood pressure, speed heart rate, and raise blood sugar levels. These changes help a person act with greater strength and speed to escape a perceived threat.

About This Chapter: This chapter includes text excerpted from "Psychological Stress And Cancer," National Cancer Institute (NCI), December 10, 2012. Reviewed October 2017.

Research has shown that people who experience intense and long-term (i.e., chronic) stress can have digestive problems, fertility problems, urinary problems, and a weakened immune system. People who experience chronic stress are also more prone to viral infections such as the flu or common cold and to have headaches, sleep trouble, depression, and anxiety.

Can Psychological Stress Cause Cancer?

Although stress can cause a number of physical health problems, the evidence that it can cause cancer is weak. Some studies have indicated a link between various psychological factors and an increased risk of developing cancer, but others have not.

Apparent links between psychological stress and cancer could arise in several ways. For example, people under stress may develop certain behaviors, such as smoking, overeating, or drinking alcohol, which increase a person's risk for cancer. Or someone who has a relative with cancer may have a higher risk for cancer because of a shared inherited risk factor, not because of the stress induced by the family member's diagnosis.

How Does Psychological Stress Affect People Who Have Cancer?

People who have cancer may find the physical, emotional, and social effects of the disease to be stressful. Those who attempt to manage their stress with risky behaviors such as smoking or drinking alcohol or who become more sedentary may have a poorer quality of life after cancer treatment. In contrast, people who are able to use effective coping strategies to deal with stress, such as relaxation and stress management techniques, have been shown to have lower levels of depression, anxiety, and symptoms related to the cancer and its treatment. However, there is no evidence that successful management of psychological stress improves cancer survival.

Evidence from experimental studies does suggest that psychological stress can affect a tumor's ability to grow and spread. For example, some studies have shown that when mice bearing human tumors were kept confined or isolated from other mice—conditions that increase stress—their tumors were more likely to grow and spread (metastasize). In one set of experiments, tumors transplanted into the mammary fat pads of mice had much higher rates of spread to the lungs and lymph nodes if the mice were chronically stressed than if the mice were not stressed. Studies in mice and in human cancer cells grown in the laboratory have found that the stress hormone norepinephrine, part of the body's fight-or-flight response system, may promote angiogenesis and metastasis.

In another study, women with triple-negative breast cancer who had been treated with neoadjuvant chemotherapy were asked about their use of beta blockers, which are medications that interfere with certain stress hormones, before and during chemotherapy. Women who reported using beta blockers had a better chance of surviving their cancer treatment without a relapse than women who did not report beta blocker use. There was no difference between the groups, however, in terms of overall survival.

Although there is still no strong evidence that stress directly affects cancer outcomes, some data do suggest that patients can develop a sense of helplessness or hopelessness when stress becomes overwhelming. This response is associated with higher rates of death, although the mechanism for this outcome is unclear. It may be that people who feel helpless or hopeless do not seek treatment when they become ill, give up prematurely on or fail to adhere to potentially helpful therapy, engage in risky behaviors such as drug use, or do not maintain a healthy lifestyle, resulting in premature death.

How Can People Who Have Cancer Learn To Cope With Psychological Stress?

Emotional and social support can help patients learn to cope with psychological stress. Such support can reduce levels of depression, anxiety, and disease- and treatment-related symptoms among patients. Approaches can include the following:

- Training in relaxation, meditation, or stress management
- Counseling or talk therapy
- Cancer education sessions
- Social support in a group setting
- Medications for depression or anxiety
- Exercise

Some expert organizations recommend that all cancer patients be screened for distress early in the course of treatment. A number also recommend rescreening at critical points along the course of care. Healthcare providers can use a variety of screening tools, such as a distress scale or questionnaire, to gauge whether cancer patients need help managing their emotions or with other practical concerns. Patients who show moderate to severe distress are typically referred to appropriate resources, such as a clinical health psychologist, social worker, chaplain, or psychiatrist.

Chapter 25

Stress And Your Developing Brain

Brain Basics

The brain is the most complex part of the human body. This three-pound organ is the seat of intelligence, interpreter of the senses, initiator of body movement, and controller of behavior. Lying in its bony shell and washed by protective fluid, the brain is the source of all the qualities that define our humanity. The brain is the crown jewel of the human body.

The Architecture Of The Brain

The brain is like a committee of experts. All the parts of the brain work together, but each part has its own special properties. The brain can be divided into three basic units: the forebrain, the midbrain, and the hindbrain.

The hindbrain includes the upper part of the spinal cord, the brain stem, and a wrinkled ball of tissue called the cerebellum. The hindbrain controls the body's vital functions such as respiration and heart rate. The cerebellum coordinates movement and is involved in learned rote movements. When you play the piano or hit a tennis ball you are activating the cerebellum. The uppermost part of the brainstem is the midbrain, which controls some reflex actions and is part of the circuit involved in the control of eye movements and other voluntary movements. The forebrain is the largest and most highly developed part of the human brain: it consists primarily of the cerebrum and the structures hidden beneath it.

About This Chapter: Text beginning with the heading "Brain Basics" is excerpted from "Brain Basics: Know Your Brain," National Institute of Neurological Disorders and Stroke (NINDS), May 19, 2017; Text beginning with the heading "How The Brain Develops" is excerpted from "Understanding The Effects Of Maltreatment On Brain Development," Child Welfare Information Gateway, U.S. Department of Health and Human Services (HHS), April 2015.

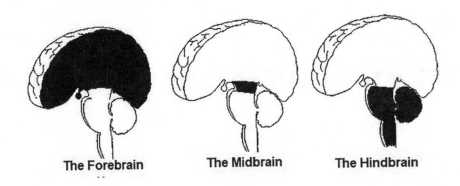

The Forebrain   The Midbrain   The Hindbrain

Figure 25.1. Brain Units

When people see pictures of the brain it is usually the cerebrum that they notice. The cerebrum sits at the topmost part of the brain and is the source of intellectual activities. It holds your memories, allows you to plan, enables you to imagine and think. It allows you to recognize friends, read books, and play games.

The cerebrum is split into two halves (hemispheres) by a deep fissure. Despite the split, the two cerebral hemispheres communicate with each other through a thick tract of nerve fibers that lies at the base of this fissure. Although the two hemispheres seem to be mirror images of each other, they are different. For instance, the ability to form words seems to lie primarily in the left hemisphere, while the right hemisphere seems to control many abstract reasoning skills.

For some as-yet-unknown reason, nearly all of the signals from the brain to the body and vice-versa crossover on their way to and from the brain. This means that the right cerebral hemisphere primarily controls the left side of the body and the left hemisphere primarily controls the right side. When one side of the brain is damaged, the opposite side of the body is affected. For example, a stroke in the right hemisphere of the brain can leave the left arm and leg paralyzed.

How The Brain Develops

What we have learned about the process of brain development helps us understand more about the roles both genetics and the environment play in our development. It appears that genetics predispose us to develop in certain ways, but our experiences, including our interactions with other people, have a significant impact on how our predispositions are expressed. In fact, research now shows that many capacities thought to be fixed at birth are actually dependent on a sequence of experiences combined with heredity. Both factors are essential for optimum development of the human brain.

Early Brain Development

The raw material of the brain is the nerve cell, called the neuron. During fetal development, neurons are created and migrate to form the various parts of the brain. As neurons migrate, they also differentiate, or specialize, to govern specific functions in the body in response to chemical signals. This process of development occurs sequentially from the "bottom up," that is, from areas of the brain controlling the most primitive functions of the body (e.g., heart rate, breathing) to the most sophisticated functions (e.g., complex thought). The first areas of the brain to fully develop are the brainstem and midbrain; they govern the bodily functions necessary for life, called the autonomic functions. At birth, these lower portions of the nervous system are very well developed, whereas the higher regions (the limbic system and cerebral cortex) are still rather primitive. Higher function brain regions involved in regulating emotions, language, and abstract thought grow rapidly in the first 3 years of life.

The Growing Child's Brain

Brain development, or learning, is actually the process of creating, strengthening, and discarding connections among the neurons; these connections are called synapses. Synapses organize the brain by forming pathways that connect the parts of the brain governing everything we do—from breathing and sleeping to thinking and feeling. This is the essence of postnatal brain development, because at birth, very few synapses have been formed. The synapses present at birth are primarily those that govern our bodily functions such as heart rate, breathing, eating, and sleeping. The development of synapses occurs at an astounding rate during a child's early years in response to that child's experiences. At its peak, the cerebral cortex of a healthy toddler may create 2 million synapses per second. By the time children are 2 years old, their brains have approximately 100 trillion synapses, many more than they will ever need. Based on the child's experiences, some synapses are strengthened and remain intact, but many are gradually discarded. This process of synapse elimination—or pruning—is a normal part of development. By the time children reach adolescence, about half of their synapses have been discarded, leaving the number they will have for most of the rest of their lives.

Another important process that takes place in the developing brain is myelination. Myelin is the white fatty tissue that forms a sheath to insulate mature brain cells, thus ensuring clear transmission of neurotransmitters across synapses. Young children process information slowly because their brain cells lack the myelin necessary for fast, clear nerve impulse transmission. Like other neuronal growth processes, myelination begins in the primary motor and sensory areas (the brainstem and cortex) and gradually progresses to the higher-order regions that control thought, memories, and feelings. Also, like other neuronal growth processes, a child's experiences affect the rate and growth of myelination, which continues into young adulthood. By 3 years of age, a baby's brain has reached almost 90 percent of its adult size. The growth in each region of the brain largely depends on receiving stimulation, which spurs activity in that region. This simulation provides the foundation for learning.

The Changing Brain And Behavior In Teens

One interpretation of all these findings is that in teens, the parts of the brain involved in emotional responses are fully online, or even more active than in adults, while the parts of the brain involved in keeping emotional, impulsive responses in check are still reaching maturity. Such a changing balance might provide clues to a youthful appetite for novelty, and a tendency to act on impulse—without regard for risk.

While much is being learned about the teen brain, it is not yet possible to know to what extent a particular behavior or ability is the result of a feature of brain structure—or a change in brain structure. Changes in the brain take place in the context of many other factors, among them, inborn traits, personal history, family, friends, community, and culture.

(Source: "The Teen Brain: Still Under Construction," National Institute of Mental Health (NIMH).)

Adolescent Brain Development

Studies using magnetic resonance imaging (MRI) techniques show that the brain continues to grow and develop into young adulthood (at least to the mid-twenties). White matter, or brain tissue, volume has been shown to increase in adults as old as 32. Right before puberty, adolescent brains experience a growth spurt that occurs mainly in the frontal lobe, which is the area that governs planning, impulse control, and reasoning. During the teenage years, the brain goes through a process of pruning synapses—somewhat like the infant and toddler brain—and also sees an increase in white matter and changes to neurotransmitter systems.

As the teenager grows into young adulthood, the brain develops more myelin to insulate the nerve fibers and speed neural processing, and this myelination occurs last in the frontal lobe. Magnetic resonance imaging (MRI) comparisons between the brains of teenagers and the brains of young adults have shown that most of the brain areas were the same—that is, the teenage brain had reached maturity in the areas that govern such abilities as speech and The major difference was the immaturity of the teenage brain in the frontal lobe and in the myelination of that area. Normal puberty and adolescence lead to the maturation of a physical body, but the brain lags behind in development, especially in the areas that allow teenagers to reason and think logically. Most teenagers act impulsively at times, using a lower area of their brains—their "gut reaction"—because their frontal lobes are not yet mature.

Impulsive behavior, poor decisions, and increased risk-taking are all part of the normal teenage experience. Another change that happens during adolescence is the growth and transformation of the limbic system, which is responsible for our emotions. Teenagers may rely on their more primitive limbic system in interpreting emotions and reacting since they lack the more mature cortex that can override the limbic response sensory capabilities.

Plasticity—The Influence Of Environment

Researchers use the term plasticity to describe the brain's ability to change in response to repeated stimulation. The extent of a brain's plasticity is dependent on the stage of development and the particular brain system or region affected. For instance, the lower parts of the brain, which control basic functions such as breathing and heart rate, are less flexible, or plastic, than the higher functioning cortex, which controls thoughts and feelings. While cortex plasticity decreases as a child gets older, some degree of plasticity remains. In fact, this brain plasticity is what allows us to keep learning into adulthood and throughout our lives. The developing brain's ongoing adaptations are the result of both genetics and experience.

Our brains prepare us to expect certain experiences by forming the pathways needed to respond to those experiences. For example, our brains are "wired" to respond to the sound of speech; when babies hear people speaking, the neural systems in their brains responsible for speech and language receive the necessary stimulation to organize and function. The more babies are exposed to people speaking, the stronger their related synapses become. If the appropriate exposure does not happen, the pathways developed in anticipation may be discarded. This is sometimes referred to as the concept of "use it or lose it." It is through these processes of creating, strengthening, and discarding synapses that our brains adapt to our unique environment. The ability to adapt to our environment is a part of normal development.

Children growing up in cold climates, on rural farms, or in large sibling groups learn how to function in those environments. Regardless of the general environment, though, all children need stimulation and nurturance for healthy development. If these are lacking (e.g., if a child's caretakers are indifferent, hostile, depressed, or cognitively impaired), the child's brain development may be impaired. Because the brain adapts to its environment, it will adapt to a negative environment just as readily as it will adapt to a positive one.

Teens And The Brain: More Questions For Research

Scientists continue to investigate the development of the brain and the relationship between the changes taking place, behavior, and health. The following questions are among the important ones that are targets of research:

How do experience and environment interact with genetic preprogramming to shape the maturing brain, and as a result, future abilities and behavior? In other words, to what extent does what a teen does and learns shape his or her brain over the rest of a lifetime?

In what ways do features unique to the teen brain play a role in the high rates of illicit substance use and alcohol abuse in the late teen to young adult years? Does the adolescent capacity for learning make this a stage of particular vulnerability to addiction?

Why is it so often the case that, for many mental disorders, symptoms first emerge during adolescence and young adulthood?

This last question has been the central reason to study brain development from infancy to adulthood. Scientists increasingly view mental illnesses as developmental disorders that have their roots in the processes involved in how the brain matures. By studying how the circuitry of the brain develops, scientists hope to identify when and for what reasons development goes off track. Brain imaging studies have revealed distinctive variations in growth patterns of brain tissue in youth who show signs of conditions affecting mental health. Ongoing research is providing information on how genetic factors increase or reduce vulnerability to mental illness; and how experiences during infancy, childhood, and adolescence can increase the risk of mental illness or protect against it.

(Source: "The Teen Brain: Still Under Construction," National Institute of Mental Health (NIMH).)

Responding To Stress

We all experience different types of stress throughout our lives. The type of stress and the timing of that stress determine whether and how there is an impact on the brain. The National Scientific Council on the Developing Child outlines three classifications of stress:

- **Positive stress** is moderate, brief, and generally a normal part of life (e.g., entering a new child care setting). Learning to adjust to this type of stress is an essential component of healthy development.

- **Tolerable stress** includes events that have the potential to alter the developing brain negatively, but which occur infrequently and give the brain time to recover (e.g., the death of a loved one).

- **Toxic stress** includes strong, frequent, and prolonged activation of the body's stress response system (e.g., chronic neglect).

Healthy responses to typical life stressors (i.e., positive and tolerable stress events) are very complex and may change depending on individual and environmental characteristics, such as genetics, the presence of a sensitive and responsive caregiver, and past experiences. A healthy stress response involves a variety of hormone and neurochemical systems throughout the body, including the sympathetic-adrenomedullary (SAM) system, which produces adrenaline, and the hypothalamicpituitary-adrenocortical (HPA) system, which produces cortisol. Increases in adrenaline help the body engage energy stores and alter blood flow. Increases in cortisol also help the body engage energy stores and also can enhance certain types of memory and activate immune responses. In a healthy stress response, the hormonal levels will return to normal after the stressful experience has passed.

Chapter 26

Eating Disorders

People with eating disorders become so focused on eating or not eating that they really hurt their bodies. People with eating disorders also may spend a lot of time thinking about their weight or how their body looks.

Eating disorders can be very dangerous. They even can be deadly.

What Is Anorexia Nervosa?

Anorexia nervosa, often called anorexia, is a very dangerous eating disorder. In fact, it is more deadly than any other mental health condition.

> ### Fast Facts
> Eating disorders can start at any age, but they usually start during the teen years. Females are more likely to get eating disorders than males.

Someone with anorexia often thinks about food and limits what she eats very strictly. She may feel like she is getting control over her life by controlling her eating. But the truth is that the disease is in control.

A person with anorexia may have some or all of the following signs:

- A low body weight for her height

- A strong fear of gaining weight

About This Chapter: This chapter includes text excerpted from "Having Eating Disorders," girlshealth.gov, Office on Women's Health (OWH), March 4, 2015.

- Thoughts that she is fat even when she is very thin

- A lot of weight loss

- Excessive exercising, like making exercise more important than many other things

- Being very careful to eat only certain foods and other extreme dieting habits

- Absent or missing menstrual periods (at least three menstrual periods in a row, if she started having periods)

- Unusual physical changes such as hair all over her body and dry, yellow skin

Anorexia can cause a lot of serious problems, including weak bones, infections, seizures, and heart trouble. If you think you or someone you know may have anorexia, talk to an adult you trust.

What Is Bulimia Nervosa?

Bulimia nervosa, usually called bulimia, has two main parts. These are binge eating and purging, which is trying to make up for the binging.

Bulimia And Health Concerns

Bulimia may cause health concerns, including:

- Inflamed and sore throat
- Swollen salivary glands (in the neck and jaw area)
- Worn tooth enamel and sensitive, decaying teeth due to stomach acid
- Acid reflux disease and other gastrointestinal problems
- Intestinal distress and irritation from laxative abuse
- Severe dehydration from purging
- Electrolyte imbalance (low or high levels of sodium, calcium, potassium, and other minerals) that can lead to stroke, heart failure, or death

(Source: "Eating Disorders," Substance Abuse and Mental Health Services Administration (SAMHSA).)

Binge eating is eating an unusually large amount of food in a short time. During a binge, a person may eat really fast even though she isn't even hungry. Someone with bulimia usually feels she can't control the binging, and may feel really embarrassed about it.

Trying to make up for the binging can take different forms. Some examples include the following:

- Purging, which means trying to get rid of the food. This could include:

- Making yourself throw up

- Taking laxatives (pills or liquids that cause a bowel movement)

- Exercising a lot

- Eating very little or not at all

- Taking pills to urinate (pee) often to lose weight

Because of these behaviors, people with bulimia may not be overweight. But they often worry about what they weigh and how their body looks.

Bulimia can cause serious health problems, including damage to your throat, teeth, stomach, and heart. If you think you or someone you know may have bulimia, talk to an adult you trust.

What Is Binge Eating Disorder?

A person with binge eating disorder eats an unusually large amount of food in a short time and feels out of control during the binges. For example, the person may eat an entire bag of cookies and a whole pizza in one short sitting.

A binge eater may feel like she can't stop overeating. That's why binge eating disorder is also sometimes called compulsive overeating. Everybody overeats sometimes, but a binge eater does it often, like once a week or more.

People with binge eating disorder also may do the following:

- Eat more quickly than usual during binges

- Eat until they are uncomfortably full

- Eat when they are not at all hungry

- Eat alone because of embarrassment

- Feel disgusted, depressed, or guilty after binging

Binge eaters are often overweight or obese, because they don't do some of the things people with bulimia or anorexia do, like throw up food or diet very strictly. Binge eating can cause a lot of health problems, including conditions that come from gaining too much weight, such as diabetes and heart disease.

> ### Binge-Eating Disorder And Health Concerns
> Binge-eating disorder may cause health concerns, including:
> - Stress
> - Weight gain, obesity, or weight cycling
> - Bloating
> - Restricted food intake
> - Dehydration
> - Problems getting along with friends and family
> - Feeling underappreciated
> - Feeling dissatisfied with life
> - High blood pressure, high cholesterol, diabetes, and other medical conditions
>
> *(Source: "Eating Disorders," Substance Abuse and Mental Health Services Administration (SAMHSA).)*

How Do I Get Help For Eating Disorders

Eating disorders are real medical illnesses. They can lead to serious problems with your heart and other parts of your body. They even can lead to death.

Eating disorders are treatable. Girls with eating disorders can go on to lead full, happy lives.

Treatment for an eating disorder may include talk therapy, medicine, and nutrition counseling. Treatment depends on the type of disorder and the needs of the person who has it.

If you think you have an eating disorder, talk to your doctor or another trusted adult. You also can call or chat with a special eating disorders helpline External link. Sometimes, a person doesn't have an eating disorder, but has unhealthy dieting behaviors that can turn into an eating disorder. If that's you, get help before any problems get worse. You deserve to feel great!

If you have an eating disorder, you may feel really bad. Don't give up! You can feel better.

Chapter 27

Body Dysmorphic Disorder

What Is Body Dysmorphic Disorder (BDD)?

Body dysmorphic disorder (BDD) is a severe, often chronic, and common disorder consisting of distressing or impairing preoccupation with perceived defects in one's physical appearance. Individuals with BDD have very poor psychosocial functioning and high rates of hospitalization and suicidality. Because BDD differs in important ways from other disorders, psychotherapies for other disorders are not adequate for BDD. Despite BDD's severity, there is no adequately tested psychosocial treatment (psychotherapy) of any type for this disorder.

Symptoms Of BDD

- Being preoccupied with minor or imaginary physical flaws, usually of the skin, hair, and nose, such as acne, scarring, facial lines, marks, pale skin, thinning hair, excessive body hair, large nose, or crooked nose.

- Having a lot of anxiety and stress about the perceived flaw and spending a lot of time focusing on it, such as frequently picking at skin, excessively checking appearance in a mirror, hiding the imperfection, comparing appearance with others, excessively grooming, seeking reassurance from others about how they look, and getting cosmetic surgery.

About This Chapter: Text under the heading "What Is Body Dysmorphic Disorder (BDD)?" is excerpted from "Cognitive-Behavioral Therapy And Supportive Psychotherapy For Body Dysmorphic Disorder," ClinicalTrials. gov, National Institutes of Health (NIH), March 15, 2016; Text beginning with the heading "Symptoms Of BDD" is excerpted from "Body Image—Cosmetic Surgery," Office on Women's Health (OWH), U.S. Department of Health and Human Services (HHS), September 22, 2009. Reviewed October 2017.

Getting cosmetic surgery can make BDD worse. They are often not happy with the outcome of the surgery. If they are, they may start to focus attention on another body area and become preoccupied trying to fix the new "defect." In this case, some patients with BDD become angry at the surgeon for making their appearance worse and may even become violent towards the surgeon.

Treatment For BDD

- **Medications.** Serotonin reuptake inhibitors or SSRIs are antidepressants that decrease the obsessive and compulsive behaviors.

- **Cognitive behavioral therapy.** This is a type of therapy with several steps:

  - The therapist asks the patient to enter social situations without covering up her "defect."

  - The therapist helps the patient stop doing the compulsive behaviors to check the defect or cover it up. This may include removing mirrors, covering skin areas that the patient picks, or not using make-up.

  - The therapist helps the patient change their false beliefs about their appearance.

Chapter 28

Self-Injury

Self-harm, sometimes called self-injury, is when a person purposely hurts his or her own body. There are many types of self-injury, and cutting is one type that you may have heard about. If you are hurting yourself, you can learn to stop. Make sure you talk to an adult you trust.

What Are Ways People Hurt Themselves?

Some types of injury leave permanent scars or cause serious health problems, sometimes even death. These are some forms of self-injury:

- Cutting yourself (such as using a razorblade, knife, or other sharp object)

- Punching yourself or punching things (like a wall)

- Burning yourself with cigarettes, matches, or candles

- Pulling out your hair

- Poking objects into body openings

- Breaking your bones or bruising yourself

- Poisoning yourself

About This Chapter: This chapter includes text excerpted from "Cutting And Self-Harm," girlshealth.gov, Office on Women's Health (OWH), January 7, 2015.

The Dangers Of Self-Injury

Some teens think self-injury is not a big deal, but it is. Self-injury comes with many risks. For example, cutting can lead to infections, scars, and even death. Sharing tools for cutting puts a person at risk of diseases like HIV and hepatitis. Also, once you start self-injuring, it may be hard to stop. And teens who keep hurting themselves are less likely to learn how to deal with their feelings in healthy ways.

Who Hurts Themselves?

People from all different kinds of backgrounds hurt themselves. Among teens, girls may be more likely to do it than boys. People of all ages hurt themselves, too, but self-injury most often starts in the teen years. People who hurt themselves sometimes have other problems like depression, eating disorders, or drug or alcohol abuse.

Why Do Some Teens Hurt Themselves?

Some teens who hurt themselves keep their feelings bottled up inside. The physical pain then offers a sense of relief, like the feelings are getting out. Some people who hold back strong emotions begin to feel like they have no emotions, and the injury helps them at least feel something.

Some teens say that when they hurt themselves, they are trying to stop feeling painful emotions, like rage, loneliness, or hopelessness. They may injure to distract themselves from the emotional pain. Or they may be trying to feel some sense of control over what they feel.

If you are depressed, angry, or having a hard time coping, talk with an adult you trust. Remember, you have a right to be safe and happy!

If you are hurting yourself, please get help. It is possible to get past the urge to hurt yourself. There are other ways to deal with your feelings. You can talk to your parents, your doctor, or another trusted adult, like a teacher or religious leader. Therapy can help you find healthy ways to handle problems.

What Are Signs Of Self-Injury In Others?

- Having cuts, bruises, or scars

- Wearing long sleeves or pants even in hot weather

- Making excuses about injuries

- Having sharp objects around for no clear reason

How Can I Help A Friend Who Is Self-Injuring?

If you think a friend may be hurting herself, try to get your friend to talk to a trusted adult. Your friend may need professional help. A therapist can suggest ways to cope with problems without turning to self-injury. If your friend won't get help, you should talk to an adult. This is too much for you to handle alone.

What If Someone Pressures Me To Hurt Myself?

If someone pressures you to hurt yourself, think about whether you really want a friend who tries to cause you pain. Try to hang out with other people who don't treat you this way. Try to hang out with people who make you feel good about yourself.

Chapter 29

Loss And Grief

Grief is defined as the primarily emotional/affective process of reacting to the loss of a loved one through death. The focus is on the internal, intrapsychic process of the individual. Normal or common grief reactions may include components such as the following:

- Numbness and disbelief.

- Anxiety from the distress of separation.

- A process of mourning often accompanied by symptoms of depression.

- Eventual recovery.

Grief reactions can also be viewed as abnormal, traumatic, pathologic, or complicated. Although no consensus has been reached, diagnostic criteria for complicated grief have been proposed.

Types Of Grief Reactions

Many authors have proposed types of grief reactions. Research has focused on normal and complicated grief while specifying types of complicated grief and available empirical support with a focus on the characteristics of different types of dysfunction. Controversy over whether it is most accurate to think of grief as progressing in sequential stages (i.e., stage theories)

About This Chapter: Text in this chapter begins with excerpts from "Grief, Bereavement, And Coping With Loss (PDQ®)—Health Professional Version," National Cancer Institute (NCI), April 20, 2017; Text under the heading "Self-Care While Grieving" is excerpted from "Veterans Employment Toolkit—Dealing With Sadness Or Grief After A Loss," U.S. Department of Veterans Affairs (VA), September 2, 2015.

continues. Most literature attempts to distinguish between normal grief and various forms of complicated grief such as chronic grief or absent/delayed/inhibited grief.

Bereavement research has tried to identify these patterns by reviewing available empirical support while also looking for evidence that these grief reactions are unique and not simply forms of major depression, anxiety, or posttraumatic stress.

Anticipatory Grief

Anticipatory grief refers to a grief reaction that occurs in anticipation of an impending loss. Anticipatory grief is the subject of considerable concern and controversy.

The term anticipatory grief is most often used when discussing the families of dying persons, although dying individuals themselves can experience anticipatory grief. Anticipatory grief includes many of the same symptoms of grief after a loss. Anticipatory grief has been defined as "the total set of cognitive, affective, cultural, and social reactions to expected death felt by the patient and family."

The following aspects of anticipatory grief have been identified among survivors:

- Depression.

- Heightened concern for the dying person.

- Rehearsal of the death.

- Attempts to adjust to the consequences of the death.

Normal Or Common Grief

In general, normal or common grief reactions are marked by a gradual movement toward an acceptance of the loss and, although daily functioning can be very difficult, managing to continue with basic daily activities. Normal grief usually includes some common emotional reactions that include emotional numbness, shock, disbelief, and/or denial often occurring immediately after the death, particularly if the death is unexpected. Much emotional distress is focused on the anxiety of separation from the loved one, which often results in yearning, searching, preoccupation with the loved one, and frequent intrusive images of death.

Over time, most bereaved people will experience symptoms less frequently, with briefer duration, or with less intensity. Although there is no clear agreement on any specific time period needed for recovery, most bereaved persons experiencing normal grief will note a lessening of symptoms at anywhere from 6 months through 2 years postloss. Normal or common grief appears to occur in 50 percent to 85 percent of persons following a loss, is time-limited, begins soon after a loss, and largely resolves within the first year or two.

Stage Models Of Normal Grief

A number of theoretically derived stage models of normal grief have been proposed. Most models hypothesize a normal grief process differentiated from various types of complicated grief. Some models have organized the variety of grief-related symptoms into phases or stages, suggesting that grief is a process marked by a series of phases, with each phase consisting of predominant characteristics. One well-known stage model, focusing on the responses of terminally ill patients to awareness of their own deaths, identified the stages of denial, anger, bargaining, depression, and acceptance. Although widely used, this model has received little empirical support.

A more recent stage model of normal grief organizes psychological responses into four stages: numbness-disbelief, separation distress, depression-mourning, and recovery. Although presented as a stage model, this model explains "it is important to emphasize that the idea that grief unfolds inexorably in regular phases is an oversimplification of the highly complex personal waxing and waning of the emotional process." Bereavement researchers have found empirical support for this four-stage model, although other researchers have questioned these findings.

Patterns Of Complicated Grief

Since the time of Sigmund Freud, many authors have proposed various patterns of pathologic or complicated grief. Some proposed patterns come from extensive clinical observation supported by various theories (e.g., psychodynamic defense mechanisms and personality traits associated with patterns of attachment).

These patterns are described in comparison to normal grief and highlight variations from the normal pattern. They include descriptive labels such as the following:

- **Inhibited or absent grief**: A pattern in which persons show little evidence of the expected separation distress, seeking, yearning, or other characteristics of normal grief.

- **Delayed grief**: A pattern in which symptoms of distress, seeking, yearning, etc., occur at a much later time than is typical.

- **Chronic grief**: A pattern emphasizing prolonged duration of grief symptoms.

- **Distorted grief**: A pattern characterized by extremely intense or atypical symptoms.

Prolonged Or Complicated Grief As A Mental Disorder

The *Diagnostic and Statistical Manual for Mental Disorders, Fourth Edition,* Text Revision (DSM-IV-TR) includes bereavement as a diagnosable code to be used when bereavement is a focus of clinical attention following the death of a loved one. In current form it does not consist of formal diagnostic criteria and is generally considered a normal reaction to loss via death. In an attempt to clearly distinguish between normal grief and complicated grief, a consensus conference has developed diagnostic criteria for a mental disorder referred to as prolonged grief disorder, proposing that it be included in the next revision of the DSM.

Following are the proposed diagnostic criteria for complicated grief:

- **Criterion A**: Person has experienced the death of a significant other, and response involves three of the four following symptoms, experienced at least daily or to a marked degree:

  - Intrusive thoughts about the deceased.

  - Yearning for the deceased.

  - Searching for the deceased.

  - Excessive loneliness since the death.

- **Criterion B**: In response to the death, four of the eight following symptoms are experienced at least daily or to a marked degree:

  - Purposelessness or feelings of futility about the future.

  - Subjective sense of numbness, detachment, or absence of emotional responsiveness.

  - Difficulty acknowledging the death (e.g., disbelief).

  - Feeling that life is empty or meaningless.

  - Feeling that part of oneself has died.

  - Shattered worldview (e.g., lost sense of security, trust, control).

  - Assumption of symptoms or harmful behaviors of, or related to, the deceased person.

  - Excessive irritability, bitterness, or anger related to the death.

- **Criterion C**: The disturbance (symptoms listed) must endure for at least 6 months.

- **Criterion D**: The disturbance causes clinically significant impairment in social, occupational, or other important areas of functioning.

These criteria have not been formally adopted, and thus there is no formal diagnostic category for prolonged grief disorders in the DSM. However, these criteria help in specifying symptoms, the severity of symptoms, and how to distinguish complicated grief from normal grief.

Children And Grief

At one time, children were considered miniature adults, and their behaviors were expected to be modeled as such. Today, there is a greater awareness of developmental differences between childhood and other developmental stages in the human life cycle. Differences between the grieving process for children and the grieving process for adults are recognized. It is now believed that the real issue for grieving children is not whether they grieve, but how they exhibit their grief and mourning.

The primary difference between bereaved adults and bereaved children is that intense emotional and behavioral expressions are not continuous in children. A child's grief may appear more intermittent and briefer than that of an adult, but in fact a child's grief usually lasts longer.

The work of mourning in childhood needs to be addressed repeatedly at different developmental and chronological milestones. Because bereavement is a process that continues over time, children will revisit the loss repeatedly, especially during significant life events (e.g., going to camp, graduating from school, marrying, and experiencing the births of their own children). Children must complete the grieving process, eventually achieving resolution of grief.

Although the experience of loss is unique and highly individualized, several factors can influence a child's grief:

- Age
- Personality
- Stage of development
- Previous experiences with death
- Previous relationship with the deceased
- Environment

- Cause of death

- Patterns of interaction and communication within the family

- Stability of family life after the loss

- How the child's needs for sustained care are met

- Availability of opportunities to share and express feelings and memories

- Parental styles of coping with stress

- Availability of consistent relationships with other adults

Children do not react to loss in the same ways as adults and may not display their feelings as openly as adults do. In addition to verbal communication, grieving children may employ play, drama, art, school work, and stories. Bereaved children may not withdraw into preoccupation with thoughts of the deceased person; they often immerse themselves in activities (e.g., they may be sad one minute and then playing outside with friends the next). Families often incorrectly interpret this behavior to mean the child does not really understand or has already gotten over the death. Neither assumption may be true; children's minds protect them from thoughts and feelings that are too powerful for them to handle.

Feeling grief is normal. Every person has her own reactions to loss. Here are some reactions you might have if you are grieving:

- Strong emotions, such as sadness, anger, worry, or guilt
- Few or no feelings, like you are emotionally numb
- Crying spells or feeling like there's a lump in your throat
- Physical reactions, such as having stomach aches or not sleeping
- Spiritual reactions, like feeling disappointed in your religion or feeling even more connected to it

Grief can go on for many months, but it should lessen over time. Everyone is different, but you should expect to feel at least a little better after a couple of months. If your grief doesn't get better over time, you may need the help of a therapist. Also, you should reach out for help without waiting if you have signs of depression. These include feeling worthless, having trouble functioning in your life, or thinking about hurting yourself.

(Source: "Dealing With Loss And Grief," girlshealth.gov, Office on Women's Health (OWH).)

Grief reactions are intermittent because children cannot explore all their thoughts and feelings as rationally as adults can. Additionally, children often have difficulty articulating their feelings about grief. A grieving child's behavior may speak louder than any words he or she could speak. Strong feelings of anger and fear of abandonment or death may be evident in the behaviors of grieving children. Children often play death games as a way of working out their feelings and anxieties in a relatively safe setting. These games are familiar to the children and provide safe opportunities to express their feelings.

Self-Care While Grieving

Taking care of yourself can help you through the process of grieving. Here are some tips:

- **Let yourself grieve.**

  Take time to experience the feelings that come with the loss. Let emotions come and go. This emotional pain can be very hard, but it's a basic part of healing.

- **Talk about your experience.**

  People may not know what you're going through. Talk to people you trust, at work and home, and let them know how to support you. Find someone who will listen without judgment. This might be a family member or friend, a chaplain or other spiritual counselor, a therapist, a Veteran or a support group.

- **Keep busy.**

  Do purposeful work that is consistent with your values.

- **Exercise.**

  Any bit of exercise can help, even just going for a short walk. Make a plan to get some form of exercise daily.

- **Eat well.**

  During times of distress, your body needs good food more than ever. Good nutrition can help you feel better physically and emotionally.

- **Wait to make major decisions.**

  Loss often involves unwanted or unexpected changes. Think about taking time to grieve before making major changes, such as selling your home or changing jobs.

- **Record your thoughts in a journal.**

  If you like to write, journaling can help. But if you find you feel worse after journaling, then stop and try another way of getting out your feelings.

- **Take advantage of your spiritual or religious beliefs.**

  You may find it helpful to call upon your spiritual beliefs to cope with your loss. Prayer or services, for instance, may be helpful. You might consult with a chaplain or pastoral counselor.

- **Get professional help if needed.**

  If you find that, over a period of time, your grief continues to interfere with your ability to move forward with your life, consider seeking help.

- **You likely have strategies that you have found helpful when you experienced a loss in the past. Utilize the strategies that work best for you.**

Chapter 30

Dealing With Depression

Depression is a serious medical illness and an important public health issue. Depression is characterized by persistent sadness and sometimes irritability (particularly in children) and is one of the leading causes of disease or injury worldwide for both men and women. Depression can cause suffering for depressed individuals and can also have negative effects on their families and the communities in which they live. Depression is associated with significant healthcare needs, school problems, loss of work, and earlier mortality.

Depression

- Is associated with an increased risk for mortality from suicide as well as other causes, such as heart disease

- Is associated with lower workplace productivity and more absenteeism, which result in lower income and higher unemployment.

- Is associated with higher risk for other conditions and behaviors, including:

  - Other mental disorders (anxiety disorders, substance use disorders, eating disorders)

  - Smoking

Although effective treatments are available, many individuals with depression do not have access to treatment or do not take advantage of services. If not effectively treated, depression is likely to become a chronic disease. Just experiencing one episode of depression places an individual at a 50 percent risk for experiencing another episode, and further increases the chances of having more depression episodes in the future.

(Source: "Depression," Centers for Disease Control and Prevention (CDC).)

About This Chapter: This chapter includes text excerpted from "Health Campaigns—Depression," Federal Occupational Health (FOH), U.S. Department of Health and Human Services (HHS), October 12, 2016.

Dealing With Depression

Depression can strongly affect your life. It can drag you down, keeping you from experiencing your full potential. Most people occasionally feel "blue," while clinically depressed people can appear to be functioning normally while just beneath the surface they struggle with feelings of sadness, discouragement, and worthlessness over a prolonged period.

Moving Forward

One of the biggest problems with depression is that it robs you of the energy and motivation necessary to deal effectively with the disorder and move forward.

The first step is realizing that you are depressed. The next step is to take action—and seek help, if you need it—so that you can successfully overcome depression and move on. The most common symptoms of depression include regularly and consistently feeling:

- Sad—"down" or "blue"
- Numb or detached—feeling "empty"
- Hopeless
- Fatigued
- Worthless—low self-esteem
- Helpless

- Overwhelmed
- Pessimistic
- Nervous or anxious
- Irritable
- Restless

You, or someone you know, may have one or more of these symptoms. If depression becomes overwhelming, or if it gets in the way of living your life as fully as you would like, talk to your Employee Assistance Program (EAP), a mental health professional, or a physician to start the first steps of moving ahead—and away from depression.

Tips For Avoiding Depression

If your depression is not too serious, you may try some simple things to help avoid biochemical, emotional, and psychological factors that can contribute to the disorder.

- Get plenty of physical activity, especially aerobic activity—brisk walking, running, biking, etc.
- Get quality sleep
- Add more social activity to your week

- Find activities that get you out and make you feel good about yourself—sports teams, adult education classes, etc.

- Avoid alcohol and other recreational drug use—drugs taken to escape or to elevate your mood rather than those used for medicinal purposes

- Volunteer—this can get you "out of yourself"—not as worried about your own problems—and it can get you into a more social environment

- Reprogram negative thought patterns with positive affirmations. For example, rather than allowing a thought like "I'm never happy" or "I wish I were happier" to dominate, you can replace this thought pattern with "I deserve to be happy" and "Everything's going my way now." The affirmation will likely not seem true at first, but as you become more comfortable with the new thought pattern, you'll begin to feel less anxious about these issues.

When To Seek Professional Help

If you continue to suffer from the effects of emotional distress and feel overwhelmed by it, you should contact a professional. Here are some red flags to look out for:

- Inability to sleep

- Feeling down, hopeless, or helpless most of the time

- Concentration problems that are interfering with your work or home life

- Using tobacco, food, drugs, or alcohol to cope with difficult emotions

- Negative or self-destructive thoughts or fears that you can't control*

- Thoughts of death or suicide*

Having self-destructive behavior or thoughts, especially suicidal ones, is a symptom that needs immediate attention. If you experience such feelings and feel that you need help, call your Employee Assistance Program (EAP) or the National Suicide Prevention Lifeline's toll-free number, which is available 24 hours every day of the year: 1-800-273-8255. This service is available to everyone. You may call for yourself or for someone you care about. All calls are confidential.

Chapter 31

Suicide

Suicide In America[1]

Suicide does not discriminate. People of all genders, ages, and ethnicities can be at risk for suicide. But people most at risk tend to share certain characteristics. The main risk factors for suicide are:

- Depression, other mental disorders, or substance abuse disorder

- A prior suicide attempt

- Family history of a mental disorder or substance abuse

- Family history of suicide

- Family violence, including physical or sexual abuse

- Having guns or other firearms in the home

- Incarceration, being in prison or jail

- Being exposed to others' suicidal behavior, such as that of family members, peers, or media figures

The risk for suicidal behavior is complex. Research suggests that people who attempt suicide differ from others in many aspects of how they think, react to events, and make

About This Chapter: This chapter includes text excerpted from documents published by two public domain sources. Text under the headings marked 1 are excerpted from "Suicide In America: Frequently Asked Questions (2015)," National Institute of Mental Health (NIMH), April 2015; Text under the heading marked 2 is excerpted from "Feeling Suicidal," girlshealth.gov, Office on Women's Health (OWH), January 7, 2015.

decisions. There are differences in aspects of memory, attention, planning, and emotion, for example. These differences often occur along with disorders like depression, substance use, anxiety, and psychosis. Sometimes suicidal behavior is triggered by events such as personal loss or violence. In order to be able to detect those at risk and prevent suicide, it is crucial that we understand the role of both long-term factors—such as experiences in childhood—and more immediate factors like mental health and recent life events. Researchers are also looking at how genes can either increase risk or make someone more resilient to loss and hardships.

Many people have some of these risk factors but do not attempt suicide. Suicide is not a normal response to stress. It is, however, a sign of extreme distress, not a harmless bid for attention.

Suicide is when people direct violence at themselves with the intent to end their lives, and they die as a result of their actions. Suicide is a leading cause of death in the United States. A suicide attempt is when people harm themselves with the intent to end their lives, but they do not die as a result of their actions. Many more people survive suicide attempts than die, but they often have serious injuries. However, a suicide attempt does not always result in a physical injury.

People who attempt suicide and survive may experience serious injuries, such as broken bones, brain damage, or organ failure. These injuries may have long-term effects on their health. People who survive suicide attempts may also have depression and other mental health problems. Suicide also affects the health of others and the community. When people die by suicide, their family and friends often experience shock, anger, guilt, and depression. The medical costs and lost wages associated with suicide also take their toll on the community.

Suicide is a serious public health problem that can have lasting harmful effects on individuals, families, and communities. While its causes are complex and determined by multiple factors, the goal of suicide prevention is simple: Reduce factors that increase risk (i.e., risk factors) and increase factors that promote resilience (i.e., protective factors). Ideally, prevention addresses all levels of influence: individual, relationship, community, and societal. Effective prevention strategies are needed to promote awareness of suicide and encourage a commitment to social change.

(Source: "Violence Prevention—Suicide," Centers for Disease Control and Prevention (CDC).)

What About Gender?[1]

Men are more likely to die by suicide than women, but women are more likely to attempt suicide. Men are more likely to use deadlier methods, such as firearms or suffocation. Women are more likely than men to attempt suicide by poisoning.

What About Children?[1]

Children and young people are at risk for suicide. Suicide is the second leading cause of death for young people ages 15 to 34.

Why Do Some Teens Think About Suicide?[2]

Some teens feel so terrible and overwhelmed that they think life will never get better. Some things that may cause these feelings include:

- The death of someone close
- Having depression or other mental health issues, such as an eating disorder, ADHD, or anxiety
- Having alcohol or drug problems
- Parents getting divorced
- Seeing a lot of anger and violence at home
- Having a hard time in school
- Being bullied
- Having problems with friends
- Experiencing a trauma like being raped or abused
- Being angry or heartbroken over a relationship break-up
- Feeling like you don't belong, either in your family or with friends
- Feeling rejected because of something about you, like being gay
- Having an ongoing illness or disability
- Feeling alone
- Feeling guilty or like a burden to other people

Also, teens sometimes may feel very bad for no one clear reason. If you are suffering, know that things definitely can get better. You can learn ways to handle your feelings. You can work toward a much brighter future.

Turning to others can help you through tough times. If you don't feel a strong connection to relatives or friends, try talking to a school counselor, teacher, doctor, or another adult you trust.

Every teen feels anxiety, sadness, and confusion at some point. The important thing to remember is that life can get much better. There is always help out there for you or a friend.

How Can Suicide Be Prevented?[1]

Effective suicide prevention is based on sound research. Programs that work take into account people's risk factors and promote interventions that are appropriate to specific groups of people. For example, research has shown that mental and substance abuse disorders are risk factors for suicide. Therefore, many programs focus on treating these disorders in addition to addressing suicide risk specifically.

Psychotherapy, or "talk therapy," can effectively reduce suicide risk. One type is called cognitive behavioral therapy (CBT). CBT can help people learn new ways of dealing with stressful experiences by training them to consider alternative actions when thoughts of suicide arise.

Another type of psychotherapy called dialectical behavior therapy (DBT) has been shown to reduce the rate of suicide among people with borderline personality disorder, a serious mental illness characterized by unstable moods, relationships, self-image, and behavior. A therapist trained in DBT helps a person recognize when his or her feelings or actions are disruptive or unhealthy, and teaches the skills needed to deal better with upsetting situations.

Medications may also help; promising medications and psychosocial treatments for suicidal people are being tested.

Still other research has found that many older adults and women who die by suicide saw their primary care providers in the year before death. Training doctors to recognize signs that a person may be considering suicide may help prevent even more suicides.

What Should I Do If Someone I Know Is Considering Suicide?[1]

If you know someone who is considering suicide, do not leave him or her alone. Try to get your loved one to seek immediate help from his or her doctor or the nearest hospital emergency room, or call 911. Remove any access he or she may have to firearms or other potential tools for suicide, including medications.

If You Are In Crisis[1]

Call the toll-free National Suicide Prevention Lifeline at 1-800-273-8255, available 24 hours a day, 7 days a week. The service is available to anyone. All calls are confidential.

What If Someone I Know Attempts Or Dies By Suicide?[1]

If someone you know attempts or dies by suicide, you may feel like it's your fault in some way. That's not true! You also may feel many different emotions, including anger, grief, or even emotional numbness. All of your feelings are okay. There is not a right or wrong way to feel.

If you are having trouble dealing with your feelings, talk to a trusted adult. You have suffered a terrible loss, but life can feel okay again. Reach out to people who care about you. Connecting is so important at this tough time.

Part Four
Diseases And Disorders With A Possible Stress Component

Chapter 32

Asthma

Depression And Asthma

Asthma and depression are both common health concerns among adolescents. For example, more than 1 in 12 adolescents have asthma. Data from the 2005 to 2014 National Survey on Drug Use and Health (NSDUH) shows that about 1 in 11 adolescents aged 12 to 17 had a major depressive episode (MDE) in the past year. MDE among adolescents is defined a period of at least 2 weeks during which they had either depressed mood or loss of interest in usual activities and also experienced a change in functioning, such as problems with sleep, eating, energy, concentration, and self-worth.2 According to 2005 to 2014 NSDUH data, adolescents aged 12 to 17 with past year asthma were more likely to have past year MDE compared to those without asthma (11.4 vs. 8.8 percent). This pattern held true among adolescents aged 12-13, 14-15 and 16-17. For example, among 16-17 year olds, those with asthma were more likely to have past year MDE than those without asthma (14.7 vs. 11.5 percent).

Assessing the relationship between asthma and depression is complicated because NSDUH data do not identify which health concern came first. Having asthma may increase the likelihood of developing depressive symptoms, while depression may impact the severity of asthma. Recognizing the association between asthma and depression among adolescents may inform prevention and treatment efforts. For example, understanding this relationship may help parents, schools, and pediatric care providers detect and start treatment.

About This Chapter: Text under the heading "Depression And Asthma" is excerpted from "The CBHSQ Report," Substance Abuse and Mental Health Services Administration (SAMHSA), May 4, 2017; Text beginning with the heading "What Is Asthma?" is excerpted from "Managing Asthma," *NIH News in Health*, National Institutes of Health (NIH), June 2014. Reviewed October 2017.

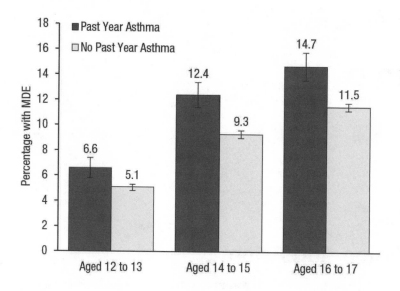

Figure 32.1. Major Depressive Episodes Among Adolescents Aged 12 To 17 (2017)

What Is Asthma?

Asthma is a common, long-lasting disease that affects the lungs. It can begin in childhood or adulthood. More than 25 million Americans have asthma, including 7 million children. Without proper care, asthma can become serious, even deadly. But most people with asthma learn to manage the disease so they have few symptoms or none at all.

What Are The Symptoms Of Asthma?

Major symptoms of asthma include wheezing (a whistling sound when breathing), shortness of breath, coughing that's worse at night and early morning, and chest tightness. These symptoms arise from reactions that narrow the airways, the tubes that carry air into and out of your lungs. When symptoms flare up, it's called an asthma attack.

The airways of people with asthma are prone to inflammation, which causes the airways to swell and narrow. They become extra sensitive to certain substances that are breathed in. These are called "triggers."

Asthma triggers can worsen inflammation and cause the muscles around the airways to tighten, further shrinking air passages and making it harder to breathe. Cells in the airways might also produce excess mucus (a sticky, thick liquid), making the airways even narrower.

Common asthma triggers include cigarette smoke, air pollution, mold, house dust mites, and furry animal dander. Other asthma triggers include weather changes, exercise, stress, and respiratory infections like common colds.

"Preventing such infections is important," stresses Dr. Stewart Levine, an asthma expert at NIH. "People who have asthma should also obtain a flu shot, as they may be at higher risk for flu-related complications."

Asthma is one of the most common causes of chronic (long term) illness in children—and some symptoms appear more often in children than in adults. "Children have smaller airways, so if they have asthma, they tend to wheeze more often, particularly during the night," says Dr. Robert Lemanske, Jr., a pediatric asthma expert at the University of Wisconsin.

Some preschool age children frequently wheeze when they get colds but don't go on to develop chronic asthma. "But some kids start wheezing at age 3, and the problem continues," says Lemanske. "These kids also tend to be more allergic."

Watch For Signs That Your Asthma Is Getting Worse

Your asthma might be getting worse if:

- Your symptoms start to occur more often, are more severe, or bother you at night and cause you to lose sleep.
- You're limiting your normal activities and missing school or work because of your asthma.
- Your peak flow number is low compared to your personal best or varies a lot from day to day.
- Your asthma medicines don't seem to work well anymore.
- You have to use your quick-relief inhaler more often. If you're using quick-relief medicine more than 2 days a week, your asthma isn't well controlled.
- You have to go to the emergency room or doctor because of an asthma attack.
- If you have any of these signs, see your doctor. He or she might need to change your medicines or take other steps to control your asthma.

(Source: "Asthma," National Heart, Lung, and Blood Institute (NHLBI).)

Diagnosis Of Asthma

A doctor will test for asthma by doing a physical exam and asking about your medical history to learn when and how often your symptoms occur. Your doctor may also ask you to breathe in and blow out into the tube of a spirometer. This device measures how much air you can breathe out and how fast you can do it.

"It's sometimes tough to do a spirometry test on young children," says Dr. Michelle Freemer, an NIH asthma expert. For youngsters, a doctor will do a physical exam and may perform other tests to identify possible asthma triggers.

Treatment For Asthma

Whether you're young or older, it's important to know how to manage your asthma. Work with your doctor to develop a written asthma action plan. Your action plan should spell out the daily treatment plan to help control your asthma. This may include recommendations for medications and for avoiding exposure to your triggers. The action plan should also give specific instructions for what to do when asthma symptoms start and what actions to take if symptoms worsen, including when to seek medical attention, go to the hospital, or call an ambulance.

"Patients with asthma should have an action plan, so they know if they're getting into trouble and what to do about it," Freemer says.

For some patients, Freemer notes that a hand-held device called a peak flow meter can help you monitor your asthma. You blow into the device to measure how strongly your lungs can force air out. If the meter shows that your air flow is lower than normal, you can use your action plan to adjust your treatment.

"There are 2 main types of medicines for managing asthma: quick-relief and long-term controllers," says Levine. Quick-relief medicines—such as short-acting bronchodilator inhalers—are used to relax the muscles in the airways to make it easier to breathe within a few minutes. If exercise is an asthma trigger, doctors may recommend taking this medicine 5 to 15 minutes before exercise or strenuous activity.

Long-term control medicines—such as inhaled corticosteroids—are used every day to help control symptoms and prevent asthma attacks. "Inhaled corticosteroids are recommended as the preferred long-term control medications for most children and adults," says Freemer. "Taken daily, they help reduce inflammation to control the disease."

If young children have trouble taking inhaled medications, there are masks and other devices that can help. Some kids are given a nebulizer, a portable machine that releases medicine in a mist.

A small percentage of people with asthma have a hard time controlling their symptoms even when they take their medicines regularly. Their airways become extremely inflamed and particularly sensitive to asthma triggers. They wheeze more, wake more throughout the night, and are at greater risk for breathing failure and trips to urgent care. If your asthma is severe, see a specialist to identify the most appropriate, personalized treatment.

The underlying causes of asthma are still unclear. Researchers believe asthma is caused by a combination of your genes and environmental factors. If you have allergies or a parent who has asthma, you're at increased risk for the disease. Obesity and exposure to cigarette smoke may also raise the risk of developing asthma. NIH scientists are continuing to investigate the causes of this disease.

Researchers are also working to develop new approaches to help prevent and treat asthma. Levine's team is studying the effects of house dust mites inside the home. While exposing mice to dust mites, the researchers identified a protein in the lung that blocked the development of asthma. With further research, the finding may eventually lead to new approaches for preventing or controlling asthma symptoms in people.

If you or your loved ones have asthma, identify your triggers and try to avoid them. Monitor your symptoms, and take prescribed medications regularly.

Keep your asthma under control so you can keep living life to the fullest.

Chapter 33

Back Pain And Emotional Distress

What Is Back Pain?

Back pain can range from a dull, constant ache to a sudden, sharp pain that makes it hard to move. It can start quickly if you fall or lift something too heavy, or it can get worse slowly.

Who Gets Back Pain?

Anyone can have back pain, but some things that increase your risk are:

- Getting older. Back pain is more common the older you get. You may first have back pain when you are 30 to 40 years old.

- Poor physical fitness. Back pain is more common in people who are not fit.

- Being overweight. A diet high in calories and fat can make you gain weight. Too much weight can stress the back and cause pain.

- Heredity. Some causes of back pain, such as ankylosing spondylitis, a form of arthritis that affects the spine, can have a genetic component.

- Other diseases. Some types of arthritis and cancer can cause back pain.

- Your job. If you have to lift, push, or pull while twisting your spine, you may get back pain. If you work at a desk all day and do not sit up straight, you may also get back pain.

About This Chapter: Text beginning with the heading "What Is Back Pain?" is excerpted from "Fast Facts About Back Pain," National Institute of Arthritis and Musculoskeletal and Skin Diseases (NIAMS), November 2014. Reviewed October 2017; Text under the heading "Chronic Pain And Stress-Related Disorders" is excerpted from "Chronic Pain And PTSD: A Guide For Patients," U.S. Department of Veterans Affairs (VA), January 3, 2014. Reviewed October 2017.

- Smoking. Your body may not be able to get enough nutrients to the disks in your back if you smoke. Smoker's cough may also cause back pain. People who smoke are slow to heal, so back pain may last longer.

Another factor is race. For example, black women are two to three times more likely than white women to have part of the lower spine slip out of place.

What Are The Causes Of Back Pain?

There are many causes of back pain. Mechanical problems with the back itself can cause pain. Examples are:

- Disk breakdown
- Spasms
- Tense muscles
- Ruptured disks

Injuries from sprains, fractures, accidents, and falls can result in back pain.

Back pain can also occur with some conditions and diseases, such as:

- Scoliosis
- Spondylolisthesis
- Arthritis
- Spinal stenosis
- Pregnancy
- Kidney stones
- Infections
- Endometriosis
- Fibromyalgia

Other possible causes of back pain are infections, tumors, or stress.

Can Back Pain Be Prevented?

The best things you can do to prevent back pain are:

- Exercise often and keep your back muscles strong.

- Maintain a healthy weight or lose weight if you weigh too much. To have strong bones, you need to get enough calcium and vitamin D every day.

- Try to stand up straight and avoid heavy lifting when you can. If you do lift something heavy, bend your legs and keep your back straight.

How Is Back Pain Diagnosed?

To diagnose back pain, your doctor will take your medical history and do a physical exam. Your doctor may order other tests, such as:

- X-rays

- Magnetic resonance imaging (MRI)

- Computed tomography (CT) scan

- Blood tests

Medical tests may not show the cause of your back pain. Many times, the cause of back pain is never known. Back pain can get better even if you do not know the cause.

How Is Back Pain Treated?

Treatment for back pain depends on what kind of pain you have. Acute back pain usually gets better without any treatment, but you may want to take acetaminophen, aspirin, or ibuprofen to help ease the pain. Exercise and surgery are not usually used to treat acute back pain.

Following are some types of treatments for chronic back pain.

Hot Or Cold Packs (Or Both)

Hot or cold packs can soothe sore, stiff backs. Heat reduces muscle spasms and pain. Cold helps reduce swelling and numbs deep pain. Using hot or cold packs may relieve pain, but this treatment does not fix the cause of chronic back pain.

Exercise

Proper exercise can help ease chronic pain but should not be used for acute back pain. Your doctor or physical therapist can tell you the best types of exercise to do.

Medications

The following are the main types of medications used for back pain:

- Analgesic medications are over-the-counter drugs such as acetaminophen and aspirin or prescription pain medications.

- Topical analgesics are creams, ointments, and salves rubbed onto the skin over the site of pain.

- Nonsteroidal anti-inflammatory drugs (NSAIDs) are drugs that reduce both pain and swelling. NSAIDs include over-the-counter drugs such as ibuprofen, ketoprofen, and naproxen sodium. Your doctor may prescribe stronger NSAIDs.

- Muscle relaxants and some antidepressants may be prescribed for some types of chronic back pain, but these do not work for every type of back pain.

Behavior Changes

You can learn to lift, push, and pull with less stress on your back. Changing how you exercise, relax, and sleep can help lessen back pain. Eating a healthy diet and not smoking also help.

Injections

Your doctor may suggest steroid or numbing shots to lessen your pain.

Complementary And Alternative Medical Treatments

When back pain becomes chronic or when other treatments do not relieve it, some people try complementary and alternative treatments. The most common of these treatments are:

- Manipulation. Professionals use their hands to adjust or massage the spine or nearby tissues.

- Transcutaneous electrical nerve stimulation (TENS). A small box over the painful area sends mild electrical pulses to nerves. Studies have shown that TENS treatments are not always effective for reducing pain.

- Acupuncture. This Chinese practice uses thin needles to relieve pain and restore health. Acupuncture may be effective when used as a part of a comprehensive treatment plan for low back pain.

- Acupressure. A therapist applies pressure to certain places in the body to relieve pain. Acupressure has not been well studied for back pain.

Surgery

Most people with chronic back pain do not need surgery. It is usually used for chronic back pain if other treatments do not work. You may need surgery if you have:

- Herniated disk. When one or more of the disks that cushion the bones of the spine are damaged, the jelly-like center of the disk leaks, causing pain.

- Spinal stenosis. This condition causes the spinal canal to become narrow.

- Spondylolisthesis. This occurs when one or more bones of the spine slip out of place.

- Vertebral fractures. A fracture can be caused by a blow to the spine or by crumbling of the bone due to osteoporosis.

- Degenerative disk disease. As people age, some have disks that break down and cause severe pain.

Rarely, when back pain is caused by a tumor, an infection, or a nerve root problem called cauda equina syndrome, surgery is needed right away to ease the pain and prevent more problems.

Chronic Pain And Stress-Related Disorders

What Is Chronic Pain?

Chronic pain is when a person suffers from pain in a particular area of the body (for example, in the back or the neck) for at least three to six months. It may be as bad as, or even worse than, short-term pain, but it can feel like more of a problem because it lasts a longer time. Chronic pain lasts beyond the normal amount of time that an injury takes to heal.

Chronic pain can come from many things. Some people get chronic pain from normal wear and tear of the body or from aging. Others have chronic pain from various types of cancer, or other chronic medical illnesses. In some cases, the chronic pain may be from an injury that happened during an accident or an assault. Some chronic pain has no explanation.

What Is The Experience Of Chronic Pain Like Physically?

There are many forms of chronic pain, including pain felt in: the low back (most common); the neck; the mouth, face, and jaw (TMJ); the pelvis; or the head (e.g., tension and migraine headaches). Of course, each type of condition results in different experiences of pain.

People with chronic pain are less able to function well in daily life than those who do not suffer from chronic pain. They may have trouble with things such as walking, standing, sitting, lifting light objects, doing paperwork, standing in line at a grocery store, going shopping, or working. Many patients with chronic pain cannot work because of their pain or physical limitations.

What Is The Experience Of Chronic Pain Like Psychologically?

Research has shown that many patients who experience chronic pain (up to 100% of these patients) tend to also be diagnosed with depression. Because the pain and disability are always there and that may even become worse over time, many of them think suicide is the only way to end their pain and frustration. They think they have no control over their life. This frustration may also lead the person to use drugs or have unneeded surgery.

Chronic Pain And PTSD

Some people's chronic pain stems from a traumatic event, such as a physical or sexual assault, a motor vehicle accident, or some type of disaster. Under these circumstances the person may experience both chronic pain and PTSD. The person in pain may not even realize the connection between their pain and a traumatic event. Approximately 15 percent to 35 percent of patients with chronic pain also have PTSD. Only 2 percent of people who do not have chronic pain have PTSD. One study found that 51 percent of patients with chronic low back pain had PTSD symptoms. For people with chronic pain, the pain may actually serve as a reminder of the traumatic event, which will tend to make the PTSD even worse. Survivors of physical, psychological, or sexual abuse tend to be more at risk for developing certain types of chronic pain later in their lives.

Chapter 34

Chronic Fatigue Syndrome

What Is Chronic Fatigue Syndrome/Myalgic Encephalomyelitis (CFS/ME)?

Chronic fatigue syndrome/myalgic encephalomyelitis/(CFS/ME) is a serious, long-term illness that affects many body systems. People with CFS/ME are often not able to do their usual activities. At times, CFS/ME may confine them to bed. People with CFS/ME have overwhelming fatigue that is not improved by rest. CFS/ME may get worse after any activity, whether it's physical or mental. This symptom is known as postexertional malaise (PEM). Other symptoms can include problems with sleep, thinking and concentrating, pain, and dizziness. People with CFS/ME may not look ill. However,

- People with CFS/ME are not able to function the same way they did before they became ill.

- CFS/ME changes people's ability to do daily tasks, like taking a shower or preparing a meal.

- CFS/ME often makes it hard to keep a job, go to school, and take part in family and social life.

- CFS/ME can last for years and sometimes leads to serious disability.

- At least one in four CFS/ME patients is bed- or house-bound for long periods during their illness.

About This Chapter: This chapter includes text excerpted from "Myalgic Encephalomyelitis/Chronic Fatigue Syndrome," Centers for Disease Control and Prevention (CDC), July 3, 2017.

Anyone can get CFS/ME. While most common in people between 40 and 60 years old, the illness affects children, adolescents, and adults of all ages. Among adults, women are affected more often than men. Whites are diagnosed more than other races and ethnicities. But many people with CFS/ME have not been diagnosed, especially among minorities.

As noted in the IOM report:

- An estimated 836,000 to 2.5 million Americans suffer from CFS/ME.

- About 90 percent of people with CFS/ME have not been diagnosed.

- CFS/ME costs the U.S. economy about $17 to $24 billion annually in medical bills and lost incomes.

Some of the reasons that people with CFS/ME have not been diagnosed include limited access to healthcare and a lack of education about CFS/ME among healthcare providers.

- Most medical schools in the United States do not have CFS/ME as part of their physician training.

- The illness is often misunderstood and might not be taken seriously by some healthcare providers.

- More education for doctors and nurses is urgently needed so they are prepared to provide timely diagnosis and appropriate care for patients.

Researchers have not yet found what causes CFS/ME, and there are no specific laboratory tests to diagnose CFS/ME directly. Therefore, doctors need to consider the diagnosis of CFS/ME based on in-depth evaluation of a person's symptoms and medical history. It is also important that doctors diagnose and treat any other conditions that can cause similar symptoms. Even though there is no cure for CFS/ME, some symptoms can be treated or managed.

Possible Causes

Scientists have not yet identified what causes myalgic encephalomyelitis/chronic fatigue syndrome (CFS/ME). It is possible that CFS/ME has more than one cause, meaning that patients with CFS/ME could have illness resulting from different causes. In addition, it is possible that two or more triggers might work together to cause the illness.

Some of the areas that are being studied as possible causes of ME/CFS are:

Infections

People with CFS/ME often have their illness begin in a way that reminds them of getting the flu. This has made researchers suspect an infection may trigger CFS/ME. In addition, about one in ten people who become infected with *Epstein-Barr virus, Ross River virus,* or *Coxiella burnetti* will develop a set of symptoms that meet the criteria for CFS/ME. People with these infections who had severe symptoms are more likely than those with mild symptoms to later develop CFS/ME symptoms. But not all people with CFS/ME have had these infections.

Other infections that have been studied in connection with CFS/ME are *human herpesvirus 6, enterovirus, rubella, Candida albicans, bornaviruses, mycoplasma, and human immunodeficiency virus (HIV).* However, these infections have not been found to cause CFS/ME.

Immune System Changes

It is possible that CFS/ME is caused by a change in the person's immune system and the way it responds to infection or stress. CFS/ME shares some features of autoimmune illnesses (diseases in which the immune system attacks healthy tissues in own body, like in rheumatoid arthritis problems). For example, both CFS/ME and most autoimmune diseases are more common in women and both are characterized by increased inflammation. However, other signs of autoimmune disease, like tissue damage, are not found in patients with CFS/ME.

Scientists think that the immune system might be contributing to CFS/ME in other ways, including:

- **Chronic production of cytokines** (cytokines are proteins that are produced by the immune system and regulate behavior of other cells). Higher levels of cytokines for a prolonged period can lead to changes in the body's ability to respond to stress and might lead to the development of health conditions, including CFS/ME.

- **Low-functioning natural killer (NK) cells.** NK cells are cells of the immune system that help the body fight infections. Many patients with CFS/ME have NK cells with lower functional ability to fight infections. Studies have found that the poorer the function of NK cells in CFS/ME patients, the worse the severity of the illness. NK cell function tests are hard to do and their results are not reliable outside of research studies. Because of this problem, NK cell function testing is not yet useful for healthcare providers. Also, low NK cell function can occur in other illnesses and thus cannot be used to diagnose CFS/ME.

- **Differences in markers of T-cell activation.** T-cells are cells of the immune system that help activate and suppress immune responses to infections. If they become too active or not active enough, the immune response does not work as it should. However, not all patients with CFS/ME appear to have these differences in markers of T-cell activation.

Stress Affecting Body Chemistry

Physical or emotional stress affects the hypothalamic-pituitary-adrenal axis (HPA axis). The HPA axis is a complex network that controls our body's reaction to stress and regulates a lot of body processes such as the immune response, digestion, energy usage, and mood. This occurs through connections between two glands of the nervous system (hypothalamus and pituitary) and adrenal glands (small organs that reside on top of the kidneys). The glands release various hormones, like corticotrophin-releasing hormone (CRH), cortisol, and others. When these hormones get out of balance, many body systems and functions, like the immune response, can be negatively affected. Cortisol, also called "the stress hormone," helps to lower inflammation and calm down the immune system. Low levels of cortisol thus may lead to an increase in inflammation and chronic activation of the immune system.

Patients with CFS/ME commonly report physical or emotional stress before they become ill. Some patients with CFS/ME have lower levels of cortisol than healthy people, but their cortisol levels are still within the normal range. Therefore, doctors cannot use cortisol levels to diagnose or treat CFS/ME.

Changes In Energy Production

Scientists found differences between people with CFS/ME and healthy people in the way cells in their bodies get their energy. However, more studies are needed to figure out how these findings may be contributing to the illness.

Possible Genetic Link

Members of the same family sometimes have CFS/ME. Studies done in twins and families suggest that both genes and environment might play a role in CFS/ME. Scientists have not yet found the exact genes or other factors from the environment that may be responsible.

Symptoms

Symptoms of chronic fatigue syndrome /myalgic encephalomyelitis (CFS/ME) may appear similar to many other illnesses and there is no test to confirm CFS/ME. This makes CFS/ME difficult to diagnose. The illness can be unpredictable. Symptoms may come and go, or there may be changes in how bad they are over time.

A doctor should be able to distinguish CFS/ME from other illnesses by doing a thorough medical exam. This includes asking many questions about the patient's health history and current illness and asking about the symptoms to learn how often they occur, how bad they are, and how long they have lasted. It is also important for doctors to talk with patients about how the symptoms affect their lives.

Primary Symptoms

Also called "core" symptoms, these occur in most patients with CFS/ME. The three primary symptoms required for diagnosis are:

- Greatly lowered ability to do activities that were usual before the illness. This drop in activity level occurs along with fatigue and must last six months or longer. People with CFS/ME have fatigue that is very different from just being tired. The fatigue of CFS/ME:

  - Can be severe.

  - Is not a result of unusually difficult activity.

  - Is not relieved by sleep or rest.

  - Was not a problem before becoming ill (not life-long).

- Worsening of CFS/ME symptoms after physical or mental activity that would not have caused a problem before illness. This is known as postexertional malaise (PEM). People with CFS/ME often describe this experience as a "crash," "relapse," or "collapse." It may take days, weeks, or longer to recover from a crash. Sometimes patients may be house-bound or even completely bed-bound during crashes. People with CFS/ME may not be able to predict what will cause a crash or how long it will last. As examples:

  - Attending a child's school event may leave someone house-bound for a couple of days and not able to do needed tasks, like laundry.

  - Shopping at the grocery store may cause a physical crash that requires a nap in the car before driving home or a call for a ride home.

  - Taking a shower may leave someone with severe CFS/ME bed-bound and unable to do anything for days.

- Sleep problems. People with CFS/ME may not feel better or less tired, even after a full night of sleep. Some people with CFS/ME may have problems falling asleep or staying asleep.

In addition to these core symptoms, one of the following two symptoms is required for diagnosis:

- Problems with thinking and memory. Most people with CFS/ME have trouble thinking quickly, remembering things, and paying attention to details. Patients often say they have "brain fog" to describe this problem because they feel "stuck in a fog" and not able to think clearly.

- Worsening of symptoms while standing or sitting upright. This is called orthostatic intolerance. People with CFS/ME may be lightheaded, dizzy, weak, or faint while standing or sitting up. They may have vision changes like blurring or seeing spots.

Other Common Symptoms

Many but not all people with CFS/ME have other symptoms.

Pain is very common in people with CFS/ME. The type of pain, where it occurs, and how bad it is varies a lot. The pain people with CFS/ME feel is not caused by an injury. The most common types of pain in CFS/ME are:

- Muscle pain and aches
- Joint pain without swelling or redness
- Headaches, either new or worsening

Some people with CFS/ME may also have:

- Tender lymph nodes in the neck or armpits
- A sore throat that happens often
- Digestive issues, like irritable bowel syndrome
- Chills and night sweats
- Allergies and sensitivities to foods, odors, chemicals, or noise

Diagnosis

To diagnose chronic fatigue syndrome/myalgic encephalomyelitis (CFS/ME), a patient's doctor or healthcare provider will:

- Ask about medical history of the patient and their family

- Do a thorough physical and mental status examination

- Order blood, urine or other tests

To get a better idea about the illness, the healthcare provider will ask many questions. Questions might include:

- What are you able to do now? How does it compare to what you were able to do before?

- How long have you felt this way?

- Do you feel better after sleeping or resting?

- What makes you feel worse? What helps you feel better?

- What happens when you try to push to do activities that are now hard for you?

- Are you able to think as clearly as you did before becoming ill?

- What symptoms keep you from doing what you need or want to do?

Patients may want to keep an activity journal. This could help them remember important details during their healthcare visit.

Doctors might refer patients to see a specialist, like a neurologist, rheumatologist, or a sleep specialist, to check for other conditions that can cause similar symptoms. These specialists might find other conditions that could be treated. Patients can have other conditions and still have CFS/ME. However, getting treatment for these conditions might help patients with CFS/ME feel better.

Treatment

There is no cure or approved treatment for chronic fatigue syndrome/myalgic encephalomyelitis (CFS/ME). However, some symptoms can be treated or managed. Treating these symptoms might provide relief for some patients with CFS/ME but not others. Other strategies, like learning new ways to manage activity, can also be helpful.

Patients, their families, and healthcare providers need to work together to decide which symptom causes the most problems. This should be treated first. Patients, families, and healthcare providers should discuss the possible benefits and harms of any treatment plans, including medicines and other therapies.

Healthcare providers need to support their patients' families as they come to understand how to live with this illness. Providers and families should remember that this process might be hard on people with CFS/ME.

Symptoms that healthcare providers might try to treat are:

Sleep Problems

Patients with CFS/ME often feel less refreshed and restored after sleep than they did before they became ill. Common sleep complaints include difficulty falling or staying asleep, extreme sleepiness, intense and vivid dreaming, restless legs, and nighttime muscle spasms.

Good sleep habits are important for all people, including those with CFS/ME. Some common tips for good sleep are:

- Start a regular bedtime routine with a long, calming wind-down period.

- Go to bed at same time each night and wake up at same time each morning.

- Limit daytime naps to 30 minutes in total during the day.

- Remove all TVs, computers, phones, and gadgets from bedroom.

- Use the bed only for sleep and sex and not for other activities (avoid reading, watching TV, listening to music, or using phones).

- Control noise, light, and temperature.

- Avoid caffeine, alcohol, and large meals before bedtime.

- Avoid exercise right before going to bed. Light exercise and stretching earlier in the day, at least four hours before bedtime, might improve sleep.

When people try these techniques but are still unable to sleep, their doctor might recommend taking medicine to help with sleep. First, people should try over-the-counter sleep products. If this does not help, doctors can offer a prescription sleep medicine, starting at the smallest dose and using for the shortest possible time.

People might continue to feel unrefreshed even after the medications help them to get a full night of sleep. If so, they should consider seeing a sleep specialist. Most people with sleep disorders, like sleep apnea (brief pause in breathing during sleep) and narcolepsy (uncontrollable sleeping), respond to therapy. However, for people with CFS/ME, not all symptoms may go away.

Pain

People with CFS/ME often have deep pain in their muscles and joints. They might also have headaches (typically pressure-like) and soreness of their skin when touched.

Patients should always talk to their healthcare provider before trying any medication. Doctors may first recommend trying over-the-counter pain-relievers, like acetaminophen, aspirin, or ibuprofen. If these do not provide enough pain relief, patients may need to see a pain specialist. People with chronic pain, including those with CFS/ME, can benefit from counseling to learn new ways to deal with pain.

Other pain management methods include stretching and movement therapies, gentle massage, heat, toning exercises, and water therapy for healing. Acupuncture, when done by a licensed practitioner, might help with pain for some patients.

Depression, Stress, And Anxiety

Adjusting to a chronic, debilitating illness sometimes leads to other problems, including depression, stress, and anxiety. Many patients with CFS/ME develop depression during their illness. When present, depression or anxiety should be treated. Although treating depression or anxiety can be helpful, it is not a cure for CFS/ME.

Some people with CFS/ME might benefit from antidepressants and antianxiety medications. However, doctors should use caution in prescribing these medications. Some drugs used to treat depression have other effects that might worsen other CFS/ME symptoms and cause side effects. When healthcare providers are concerned about patient's psychological condition, they may recommend seeing a mental health professional.

Some people with CFS/ME might benefit from trying techniques like deep breathing and muscle relaxation, massage, and movement therapies (such as stretching, yoga, and tai chi). These can reduce stress and anxiety, and promote a sense of well-being.

Dizziness And Lightheadedness (Orthostatic Intolerance)

Some people with CFS/ME might also have symptoms of orthostatic intolerance that are triggered when-or made worse by-standing or sitting upright. These symptoms can include:

- Frequent dizziness and lightheadedness
- Changes in vision (blurred vision, seeing white or black spots)
- Weakness
- Feeling like your heart is beating too fast or too hard, fluttering, or skipping a beat

For patients with these symptoms, their doctor will check their heart rate and blood pressure, and may recommend they see a specialist, like a cardiologist or neurologist.

For people with CFS/ME who do not have heart or blood vessel disease, doctor might suggest patients increase daily fluid and salt intake and use support stockings. If symptoms do not improve, prescription medication can be considered.

Memory And Concentration Problems

Memory aids, like organizers and calendars, can help with memory problems. For people with CFS/ME who have concentration problems, some doctors have prescribed stimulant medications, like those typically used to treat attention deficit hyperactivity disorder (ADHD). While stimulants might help improve concentration for some patients with CFS/ME, they might lead to the 'push-and-crash' cycle and worsen symptoms. "Push-and-crash" cycles are when someone with CFS/ME is having a good day and tries to push to do more than they would normally attempt (do too much, crash, rest, start to feel a little better, do too much once again).

Strategies that do not involve use of medications and might be helpful to some patients-particularly if their illness does not keep them bed-bound-are:

- Avoiding 'push-and-crash' cycles through carefully managing activity. "Push-and-crash" cycles are when someone with CFS/ME is having a good day and tries to push to do more than they would normally attempt (do too much, crash, rest, start to feel a little better, do too much once again). This can then lead to a "crash" (worsening of CFS/ME symptoms). Finding ways to make activities easier may be helpful, like sitting while doing the laundry or showering, taking frequent breaks, and dividing large tasks into smaller steps.

- Talking with a therapist to help find strategies to cope with the illness and its impact on daily life and relationships.

Other potentially supportive treatments or strategies include:

- Balanced diet. A balanced diet is important for everyone's good health and would benefit a person with or without any chronic illness.

- Nutritional supplements. Doctors might run tests to see if patients lack any important nutrients and might suggest supplements to try. Doctors and patients should talk about any risks and benefits of supplements, and consider any possible interactions that may occur with prescription medications. Follow-up tests to see if nutrient levels improve can help with treatment planning.

- Complementary therapies. Complementary therapies, like acupuncture, meditation, gentle massage, deep breathing, relaxation therapy, yoga, or tai chi, might be helpful to increase energy and decrease pain.

Patients should talk with their doctors about all potential therapies because many treatments that are promoted as cures for CFS/ME are unproven, often costly, and could be dangerous.

Chapter 35

Fibromyalgia

What Is Fibromyalgia?

Fibromyalgia is a condition that causes pain all over the body (also referred to as widespread pain), sleep problems, fatigue, and often emotional and mental distress. People with fibromyalgia may be more sensitive to pain than people without fibromyalgia. This is called abnormal pain perception processing. Fibromyalgia affects about 4 million U.S. adults, about 2 percent of the adult population. The cause of fibromyalgia is not known, but it can be effectively treated and managed.

How Do I Know I Might Have Fibromyalgia?

The most common symptoms of fibromyalgia are:

- Pain and stiffness all over the body.

- Fatigue and tiredness.

- Depression and anxiety.

- Sleep problems.

- Problems with thinking, memory, and concentration.

- Headaches, including migraines.

About This Chapter: This chapter includes text excerpted from "Fibromyalgia," Centers for Disease Control and Prevention (CDC), May 4, 2017.

Other symptoms may include:

- Tingling or numbness in hands and feet.

- Pain in the face or jaw, including disorders of the jaw known as temporomandibular joint syndrome (also known as TMJ).

- Digestive problems, such as abdominal pain, bloating, constipation, and even irritable bowel syndrome (also known as IBS).

What Are The Risk Factors For Fibromyalgia?

Known risk factors include:

- Age. Fibromyalgia can affect people of all ages, including children. However, most people are diagnosed during middle age and you are more likely to have fibromyalgia as you get older.

- Lupus or Rheumatoid Arthritis. If you have lupus or rheumatoid arthritis (RA), you are more likely to develop fibromyalgia.

Some other factors have been weakly associated with onset of fibromyalgia, but more research is needed to see if they are real. These possible risk factors include:

- Sex. Women are twice as likely to have fibromyalgia as men.
- Stressful or traumatic events, such as car accidents, posttraumatic stress disorder (PTSD).
- Repetitive injuries. Injury from repetitive stress on a joint, such as frequent knee bending.
- Illness (such as viral infections).
- Family history.
- Obesity.

How Is Fibromyalgia Diagnosed?

Doctors usually diagnose fibromyalgia using the patient's history, physical examination, X-rays, and blood work.

How Is Fibromyalgia Treated?

Fibromyalgia can be effectively treated and managed with medication and self-management strategies. Fibromyalgia should be treated by a doctor or team of healthcare professionals who specialize in the treatment of fibromyalgia and other types of arthritis, called rheumatologists. Doctors usually treat fibromyalgia with a combination of treatments, which may include:

- Medications, including prescription drugs and over-the-counter pain relievers.

- Aerobic exercise and muscle strengthening exercise.

- Patient education classes, usually in primary care or community settings.

- Stress management techniques such as meditation, yoga, and massage.

- Good sleep habits to improve the quality of sleep.

- Cognitive behavioral therapy (CBT) to treat underlying depression. CBT is a type of talk therapy meant to change the way people act or think.

In addition to medical treatment, people can manage their fibromyalgia with the self-management strategies, which are proven to reduce pain and disability, so they can pursue the activities important to them.

What Are The Complications Of Fibromyalgia?

Fibromyalgia can cause pain, disability, and lower quality of life. U.S. adults with fibromyalgia may have complications such as:

- More hospitalizations. If you have fibromyalgia you are twice as likely to be hospitalized as someone without fibromyalgia.

- Lower quality of life. Women with fibromyalgia have low quality of life. If you're a woman with fibromyalgia you may have 40 percent less physical function and 67 percent less mental health.

- Higher rates of major depression. Adults with fibromyalgia are more than 3 times more likely to have major depression than adults without fibromyalgia. Screening and treatment for depression is extremely important.

- Higher death rates from suicide and injuries. Death rates from suicide and injuries are higher among fibromyalgia patients, but overall mortality among adults with fibromyalgia is similar to the general population.

- Higher rates of other rheumatic conditions. Fibromyalgia often co-occurs with other types of arthritis such as osteoarthritis, rheumatoid arthritis, systemic lupus erythematosus, and ankylosing spondylitis.

How Can I Improve My Quality Of Life?

- **Get physically active.** Experts recommend that adults be moderately physically active for 150 minutes per week. Walk, swim, or bike 30 minutes a day for five days a week. These 30 minutes can be broken into three separate ten-minute sessions during the day. Regular physical activity can also reduce the risk of developing other chronic diseases such as heart disease and diabetes.

- **Go to recommended physical activity programs.** Those concerned about how to safely exercise can participate in physical activity programs that are proven effective for reducing pain and disability related to arthritis and improving mood and the ability to move. Classes take place at local Ys, parks, and community centers. These classes can help you feel better.

- **Join a self-management education class,** which helps people with arthritis or other conditions—including fibromyalgia—be more confident in how to control their symptoms, how to live well and understand how the condition affects their lives.

Chapter 36

Multiple Sclerosis

What Is Multiple Sclerosis?

Multiple sclerosis (MS) is a nervous system disease that affects your brain and spinal cord. It damages the myelin sheath, the material that surrounds and protects your nerve cells. This damage slows down or blocks messages between your brain and your body, leading to the symptoms of MS. They can include:

- Visual disturbances

- Muscle weakness

- Trouble with coordination and balance

- Sensations such as numbness, prickling, or "pins and needles"

- Thinking and memory problems

No one knows what causes MS. It may be an autoimmune disease, which happens when your immune system attacks healthy cells in your body by mistake. Multiple sclerosis affects women more than men. It often begins between the ages of 20 and 40. Usually, the disease is mild, but some people lose the ability to write, speak, or walk.

There is no single test for MS. Doctors use a medical history, physical exam, neurological exam, Magnetic resonance imaging MRI, and other tests to diagnose it. There is no cure for

About This Chapter: Text under the heading "What Is Multiple Sclerosis?" is excerpted from "Multiple Sclerosis," MedlinePlus, National Institutes of Health (NIH), August 6, 2014. Reviewed October 2017; Text beginning with heading "What Are Plaques Made Of And Why Do They Develop?" is excerpted from "Multiple Sclerosis: Hope Through Research," National Institute of Neurological Disorders and Stroke (NINDS), June 2012. Reviewed October 2017.

MS, but medicines may slow it down and help control symptoms. Physical and occupational therapy may also help.

What Are Plaques Made Of And Why Do They Develop?

Plaques, or *lesions*, are the result of an inflammatory process in the brain that causes immune system cells to attack myelin. The myelin sheath helps to speed nerve impulses traveling within the nervous system. Axons are also damaged in MS, although not as extensively, or as early in the disease, as myelin.

Under normal circumstances, cells of the immune system travel in and out of the brain patrolling for infectious agents (viruses, for example) or unhealthy cells. This is called the "surveillance" function of the immune system.

Surveillance cells usually won't spring into action unless they recognize an infectious agent or unhealthy cells. When they do, they produce substances to stop the infectious agent. If they encounter unhealthy cells, they either kill them directly or clean out the dying area and produce substances that promote healing and repair among the cells that are left.

Researchers have observed that immune cells behave differently in the brains of people with MS. They become active and attack what appears to be healthy myelin. It is unclear what triggers this attack. MS is one of many *autoimmune disorders,* such as rheumatoid arthritis and lupus, in which the immune system mistakenly attacks a person's healthy tissue as opposed to performing its normal role of attacking foreign invaders like viruses and bacteria. Whatever the reason, during these periods of immune system activity, most of the myelin within the affected area is damaged or destroyed. The axons also may be damaged. The symptoms of MS depend on the severity of the immune reaction as well as the location and extent of the plaques, which primarily appear in the brain stem, cerebellum, spinal cord, optic nerves, and the white matter of the brain around the brain ventricles (fluid-filled spaces inside of the brain).

What Are The Signs And Symptoms Of MS?

The symptoms of MS usually begin over one to several days, but in some forms, they may develop more slowly. They may be mild or severe and may go away quickly or last for months. Sometimes the initial symptoms of MS are overlooked because they disappear in a day or so and normal function returns. Because symptoms come and go in the majority of people with MS, the presence of symptoms is called an attack, or in medical terms, an exacerbation.

Recovery from symptoms is referred to as remission, while a return of symptoms is called a relapse. This form of MS is therefore called relapsing-remitting MS, in contrast to a more slowly developing form called primary progressive MS. Progressive MS can also be a second stage of the illness that follows years of relapsing-remitting symptoms.

A diagnosis of MS is often delayed because MS shares symptoms with other neurological conditions and diseases.

The first symptoms of MS often include:

- vision problems such as blurred or double vision or optic neuritis, which causes pain in the eye and a rapid loss of vision.

- weak, stiff muscles, often with painful muscle spasms

- tingling or numbness in the arms, legs, trunk of the body, or face

- clumsiness, particularly difficulty staying balanced when walking

- bladder control problems, either inability to control the bladder or urgency

- dizziness that doesn't go away

MS may also cause later symptoms such as:

- mental or physical fatigue which accompanies the above symptoms during an attack

- mood changes such as depression or euphoria

- changes in the ability to concentrate or to multitask effectively

- difficulty making decisions, planning, or prioritizing at work or in private life.

Some people with MS develop *transverse myelitis,* a condition caused by inflammation in the spinal cord. Transverse myelitis causes loss of spinal cord function over a period of time lasting from several hours to several weeks. It usually begins as a sudden onset of lower back pain, muscle weakness, or abnormal sensations in the toes and feet, and can rapidly progress to more severe symptoms, including paralysis. In most cases of transverse myelitis, people recover at least some function within the first 12 weeks after an attack begins. Transverse myelitis can also result from viral infections, arteriovenous malformations, or neuroinflammatory problems unrelated to MS. In such instances, there are no plaques in the brain that suggest previous MS attacks.

Neuro-myelitis optica is a disorder associated with transverse myelitis as well as optic nerve inflammation. Patients with this disorder usually have *antibodies* against a particular protein in their spinal cord, called the aquaporin channel. These patients respond differently to treatment than most people with MS.

Most individuals with MS have muscle weakness, often in their hands and legs. Muscle stiffness and spasms can also be a problem. These symptoms may be severe enough to affect walking or standing. In some cases, MS leads to partial or complete paralysis. Many people with MS find that weakness and fatigue are worse when they have a fever or when they are exposed to heat. MS exacerbations may occur following common infections.

Tingling and burning sensations are common, as well as the opposite, numbness and loss of sensation. Moving the neck from side to side or flexing it back and forth may cause "Lhermitte sign," a characteristic sensation of MS that feels like a sharp spike of electricity coursing down the spine.

While it is rare for pain to be the first sign of MS, pain often occurs with optic neuritis and trigeminal neuralgia, a neurological disorder that affects one of the nerves that runs across the jaw, cheek, and face. Painful spasms of the limbs and sharp pain shooting down the legs or around the abdomen can also be symptoms of MS.

Most individuals with MS experience difficulties with coordination and balance at some time during the course of the disease. Some may have a continuous trembling of the head, limbs, and body, especially during movement, although such trembling is more common with other disorders such as Parkinson disease.

Fatigue is common, especially during exacerbations of MS. A person with MS may be tired all the time or may be easily fatigued from mental or physical exertion.

Urinary symptoms, including loss of bladder control and sudden attacks of urgency, are common as MS progresses. People with MS sometimes also develop constipation or sexual problems.

Depression is a common feature of MS. A small number of individuals with MS may develop more severe psychiatric disorders such as bipolar disorder and paranoia, or experience inappropriate episodes of high spirits, known as euphoria.

People with MS, especially those who have had the disease for a long time, can experience difficulty with thinking, learning, memory, and judgment. The first signs of what doctors call cognitive dysfunction may be subtle. The person may have problems finding the right word to say, or trouble remembering how to do routine tasks on the job or at home. Day-to-day decisions that once came easily may now be made more slowly and show poor judgment. Changes may be so small or happen so slowly that it takes a family member or friend to point them out.

How Many People Have MS?

No one knows exactly how many people have MS. Experts think there are 250,000 to 350,000 people in the United States diagnosed with MS. This estimate suggests that approximately 200 new cases are diagnosed every week. Studies of the prevalence (the proportion of individuals in a population having a particular disease) of MS indicate that the rate of the disease has increased steadily during the twentieth century.

As with most autoimmune disorders, twice as many women are affected by MS as men. MS is more common in colder climates. People of Northern European descent appear to be at the highest risk for the disease, regardless of where they live. Native Americans of North and South America, as well as Asian American populations, have relatively low rates of MS.

What Causes MS?

The ultimate cause of MS is damage to myelin, nerve fibers, and neurons in the brain and spinal cord, which together make up the central nervous system (CNS). But how that happens, and why, are questions that challenge researchers. Evidence appears to show that MS is a disease caused by genetic vulnerabilities combined with environmental factors.

Although there is little doubt that the immune system contributes to the brain and spinal cord tissue destruction of MS, the exact target of the immune system attacks and which immune system cells cause the destruction isn't fully understood.

Researchers have several possible explanations for what might be going on. The immune system could be:

- fighting some kind of infectious agent (for example, a virus) that has components which mimic components of the brain (molecular mimicry)

- destroying brain cells because they are unhealthy

- mistakenly identifying normal brain cells as foreign

The last possibility has been the favored explanation for many years. Research now suggests that the first two activities might also play a role in the development of MS. There is a special barrier, called the *blood-brain barrier*, which separates the brain and spinal cord from the immune system. If there is a break in the barrier, it exposes the brain to the immune system for the first time. When this happens, the immune system may misinterpret the brain as "foreign."

Genetic Susceptibility

Susceptibility to MS may be inherited. Studies of families indicate that relatives of an individual with MS have an increased risk for developing the disease. Experts estimate that about 15 percent of individuals with MS have one or more family members or relatives who also have MS. But even identical twins, whose DNA is exactly the same, have only a 1 in 3 chance of both having the disease. This suggests that MS is not entirely controlled by genes. Other factors must come into play.

Research suggests that dozens of genes and possibly hundreds of variations in the genetic code (called gene variants) combine to create vulnerability to MS. Some of these genes have been identified. Most of the genes identified so far are associated with functions of the immune system. Additionally, many of the known genes are similar to those that have been identified in people with other autoimmune diseases as type 1 diabetes, rheumatoid arthritis or lupus. Researchers continue to look for additional genes and to study how they interact with each other to make an individual vulnerable to developing MS.

Sunlight And Vitamin D

A number of studies have suggested that people who spend more time in the sun and those with relatively high levels of vitamin D are less likely to develop MS. Bright sunlight helps human skin produce vitamin D. Researchers believe that vitamin D may help regulate the immune system in ways that reduce the risk of MS. People from regions near the equator, where there is a great deal of bright sunlight, generally have a much lower risk of MS than people from temperate areas such as the United States and Canada. Other studies suggest that people with higher levels of vitamin D generally have less severe MS and fewer relapses.

Smoking

A number of studies have found that people who smoke are more likely to develop MS. People who smoke also tend to have more brain lesions and brain shrinkage than nonsmokers. The reasons for this are currently unclear.

Infectious Factors And Viruses

A number of viruses have been found in people with MS, but the virus most consistently linked to the development of MS is Epstein Barr virus (EBV), the virus that causes mononucleosis. Only about 5 percent of the population has not been infected by EBV. These individuals are at a lower risk for developing MS than those who have been infected. People who were infected with

EBV in adolescence or adulthood and who therefore develop an exaggerated immune response to EBV are at a significantly higher risk for developing MS than those who were infected in early childhood. This suggests that it may be the type of immune response to EBV that predisposes to MS, rather than EBV infection itself. However, there is still no proof that EBV causes MS.

Autoimmune And Inflammatory Processes

Tissue inflammation and antibodies in the blood that fight normal components of the body and tissue in people with MS are similar to those found in other autoimmune diseases. Along with overlapping evidence from genetic studies, these findings suggest that MS results from some kind of disturbed regulation of the immune system.

How Is MS Diagnosed?

There is no single test used to diagnose MS. Doctors use a number of tests to rule out or confirm the diagnosis. There are many other disorders that can mimic MS. Some of these other disorders can be cured, while others require different treatments than those used for MS. Therefore it is very important to perform a thorough investigation before making a diagnosis.

In addition to a complete medical history, physical examination, and a detailed neurological examination, a doctor will order an MRI scan of the head and spine to look for the characteristic lesions of MS. MRI is used to generate images of the brain and/or spinal cord. Then a special dye or contrast agent is injected into a vein and the MRI is repeated. In regions with active inflammation in MS, there is disruption of the blood-brain barrier and the dye will leak into the active MS lesion.

Doctors may also order evoked potential tests, which use electrodes on the skin and painless electric signals to measure how quickly and accurately the nervous system responds to stimulation. In addition, they may request a lumbar puncture (sometimes called a "spinal tap") to obtain a sample of *cerebrospinal fluid*. This allows them to look for proteins and inflammatory cells associated with the disease and to rule out other diseases that may look similar to MS, including some infections and other illnesses. MS is confirmed when positive signs of the disease are found in different parts of the nervous system at more than one time interval and there is no alternative diagnosis.

What Is The Course Of MS?

The course of MS is different for each individual, which makes it difficult to predict. For most people, it starts with a first attack, usually (but not always) followed by a full to almost-full recovery. Weeks, months, or even years may pass before another attack occurs, followed again by a period of relief from symptoms. This characteristic pattern is called relapsing-remitting MS.

Primary-progressive MS is characterized by a gradual physical decline with no noticeable remissions, although there may be temporary or minor relief from symptoms. This type of MS has a later onset, usually after age 40, and is just as common in men as in women.

Secondary-progressive MS begins with a relapsing-remitting course, followed by a later primary-progressive course. The majority of individuals with severe relapsing-remitting MS will develop secondary progressive MS if they are untreated.

Finally, there are some rare and unusual variants of MS. One of these is Marburg variant MS (also called malignant MS), which causes a swift and relentless decline resulting in significant disability or even death shortly after disease onset. Balo's concentric sclerosis, which causes concentric rings of demyelination that can be seen on an MRI, is another variant type of MS that can progress rapidly.

Determining the particular type of MS is important because the current disease modifying drugs have been proven beneficial only for the relapsing-remitting types of MS.

What Is An Exacerbation Or Attack Of MS?

An exacerbation—which is also called a relapse, flare-up, or attack—is a sudden worsening of MS symptoms, or the appearance of new symptoms that lasts for at least 24 hours. MS relapses are thought to be associated with the development of new areas of damage in the brain. Exacerbations are characteristic of relapsing-remitting MS, in which attacks are followed by periods of complete or partial recovery with no apparent worsening of symptoms.

An attack may be mild or its symptoms may be severe enough to significantly interfere with life's daily activities. Most exacerbations last from several days to several weeks, although some have been known to last for months.

When the symptoms of the attack subside, an individual with MS is said to be in remission. However, MRI data have shown that this is somewhat misleading because MS lesions continue to appear during these remission periods. Patients do not experience symptoms during remission because the inflammation may not be severe or it may occur in areas of the brain that do not produce obvious symptoms. Research suggests that only about 1 out of every 10 MS lesions is perceived by a person with MS. Therefore, MRI examination plays a very important role in establishing an MS diagnosis, deciding when the disease should be treated, and determining whether treatments work effectively or not. It also has been a valuable tool to test whether an experimental new therapy is effective at reducing exacerbations.

Are There Treatments Available For MS?

There is still no cure for MS, but there are treatments for initial attacks, medications and therapies to improve symptoms, and recently developed drugs to slow the worsening of the disease. These new drugs have been shown to reduce the number and severity of relapses and to delay the long-term progression of MS.

Treatments For Attacks

The usual treatment for an initial MS attack is to inject high doses of a steroid drug, such as methylprednisolone, intravenously (into a vein) over the course of 3 to 5 days. It may sometimes be followed by a tapered dose of oral steroids. Intravenous steroids quickly and potently suppress the immune system, and reduce inflammation. Clinical trials have shown that these drugs hasten recovery.

The American Academy of Neurology (AAN) recommends using *plasma* exchange as a secondary treatment for severe flare-ups in relapsing forms of MS when the patient does not have a good response to methylprednisolone. Plasma exchange, also known as *plasmapheresis,* involves taking blood out of the body and removing components in the blood's plasma that are thought to be harmful. The rest of the blood, plus replacement plasma, is then transfused back into the body. This treatment has not been shown to be effective for secondary progressive or chronic progressive forms of MS.

Treatments To Help Reduce Disease Activity And Progression

During the past 20 years, researchers have made major breakthroughs in MS treatment due to new knowledge about the immune system and the ability to use MRI to monitor MS in patients. As a result, a number of medical therapies have been found to reduce relapses in persons with relapsing-remitting MS. These drugs are called disease modulating drugs.

There is debate among doctors about whether to start disease modulating drugs at the first signs of MS or to wait until the course of the disease is better defined before beginning treatment. On one hand, U.S. Food and Drug Administration (FDA)-approved medications to treat MS work best early in the course of the disease and work poorly, if at all, later in the progressive phase of the illness. Clinical trials have shown convincingly that delaying treatment, even for the 1 to-2 years that it may take for patients with MS to develop a second clinical attack, may lead to an irreversible increase in disability. In addition, people who begin treatment after their first attack have fewer brain lesions and fewer relapses over time.

On the other hand, initiating treatment in patients with a single attack and no signs of previous MS lesions, before MS is diagnosed, poses risks because all FDA-approved medications to treat MS are associated with some side effects. Therefore, the best strategy is to have a thorough diagnostic work-up at the time of first attack of MS. The work-up should exclude all other diseases that can mimic MS so that the diagnosis can be determined with a high probability. The diagnostic tests may include an evaluation of the cerebrospinal fluid and repeated MRI examinations. If such a thorough work-up cannot confirm the diagnosis of MS with certainty, it may be prudent to wait before starting treatment. However, each patient should have a scheduled follow-up evaluation by his or her neurologist 6 to 12 months after the initial diagnostic evaluation, even in the absence of any new attacks of the disease. Ideally, this evaluation should include an MRI examination to see if any new MS lesions have developed without causing symptoms.

Until recently, it appeared that a minority of people with MS had very mild disease or "benign MS" and would never get worse or become disabled. This group makes up 10 to 20 percent of those with MS. Doctors were concerned about exposing such benign MS patients to the side effects of MS drugs. However, recent data from the long-term follow-up of these patients indicate that after 10 to 20 years, some of these patients become disabled. Therefore, current evidence supports discussing the start of therapy early with all people who have MS, as long as the MS diagnosis has been thoroughly investigated and confirmed. There is an additional small group of individuals (approximately 1 percent) whose course will progress so rapidly that they will require aggressive and perhaps even experimental treatment.

FDA-approved therapies for MS are designed to modulate or suppress the inflammatory reactions of the disease. They are most effective for relapsing-remitting MS at early stages of the disease. These treatments include injectable beta interferon drugs. Interferons are signaling molecules that regulate immune cells. Potential side effects of beta interferon drugs include flu-like symptoms, such as fever, chills, muscle aches, and fatigue, which usually fade with continued therapy. A few individuals will notice a decrease in the effectiveness of the drugs after 18 to 24 months of treatment due to the development of antibodies that neutralize the drugs' effectiveness. If the person has flare-ups or worsening symptoms, doctors may switch treatment to alternative drugs.

Glatiramer acetate is another injectable immune-modulating drug used for MS. Exactly how it works is not entirely clear, but research has shown that it changes the balance of immune cells in the body. Side effects with glatiramer acetate are usually mild, but it can cause skin reactions and allergic reactions. It is approved only for relapsing forms of MS.

The drug mitoxantrone, which is administered intravenously four times a year, has been approved for especially severe forms of relapsing-remitting and secondary progressive MS. This drug has been associated with development of certain types of blood cancers in up to one percent of patients, as well as with heart damage. Therefore, this drug should be used as a last resort to treat patients with a form of MS that leads to rapid loss of function and for whom other treatments did not stop the disease.

Natalizumab works by preventing cells of the immune system from entering the brain and spinal cord. It is administered intravenously once a month. It is a very effective drug for many people, but it is associated with an increased risk of a potentially fatal viral infection of the brain called progressive multifocal encephalopathy (PML). People who take natalizumab must be carefully monitored for symptoms of PML, which include changes in vision, speech, and balance that do not remit like an MS attack. Therefore, natalizumab is generally recommended only for individuals who have not responded well to the other approved MS therapies or who are unable to tolerate them. Other side effects of natalizumab treatment include allergic and hypersensitivity reactions.

In 2010, the FDA approved fingolimod, the first MS drug that can be taken orally as a pill, to treat relapsing forms of MS. The drug prevents white blood cells called lymphocytes from leaving the lymph nodes and entering the blood and the brain and spinal cord. The decreased number of lymphocytes in the blood can make people taking fingolimod more susceptible to infections. The drug may also cause problems with eyes and with blood pressure and heart rate. Because of this, the drug must be administered in a doctor's office for the first time and the

Table 36.1. Disease Modifying Drugs

Trade Name	Generic Name
Avonex	interferon beta-1a
Betaseron	interferon beta-1b
Rebif	interferon beta-1a
Copaxone	glatiramer acetate
Tysabri	natalizumab
Novantrone	mitoxantrone
Gilenya	fingolimod

treating physician must evaluate the patient's vision and blood pressure during an early follow-up examination. The exact frequency of rare side effects (such as severe infections) of fingolimod is unknown. In March 2017, the FDA approved ocrelizumab (brand name Ocrevus) to treat adults with relapsing forms of MS and primary progressive multiple sclerosis.

Other FDA-approved drugs to treat relapsing forms of MS in adults include dimethyl fumarate and teriflunomide, both taken orally.

Chapter 37

Lupus

If you have lupus, you probably have many questions. Lupus isn't a simple disease with an easy answer. You can't take a pill and make it go away. The people you live with and work with may have trouble understanding that you're sick. Lupus doesn't have a clear set of signs that people can see. You may know that something's wrong, even though it may take a while to be diagnosed.

Lupus has many shades. It can affect people of different races, ethnicities, and ages, both men and women. It can look like different diseases. It's different for every person who has it. The good news is that you can get help and fight lupus. Learning about it is the first step. Ask questions. Talk to your doctor, family, and friends. People who look for answers are more likely to find them. This chapter can help you get started.

What Is Lupus?

Lupus is an autoimmune disease. Your body's immune system is like an army with hundreds of soldiers. The immune system's job is to fight foreign substances in the body, like germs and viruses. But in autoimmune diseases, the immune system is out of control. It attacks healthy tissues, not germs.

You can't catch lupus from another person. It isn't cancer, and it isn't related to acquired immunodeficiency syndrome (AIDS). Lupus is a disease that can affect many parts of the body. Everyone reacts differently. One person with lupus may have swollen knees and fever. Another person may be tired all the time or have kidney trouble. Someone else may have

About This Chapter: This chapter includes text excerpted from "Living With Lupus: Health Information Basics For You And Your Family," National Institute of Arthritis and Musculoskeletal and Skin Diseases (NIAMS), April 2017.

rashes. Lupus can involve the joints, the skin, the kidneys, the lungs, the heart, and/or the brain. If you have lupus, it may affect two or three parts of your body. Usually, one person doesn't have all the possible symptoms.

There are three main types of lupus:

- **Systemic lupus erythematosus** is the most common form. It's sometimes called SLE, or just lupus. The word "systemic" means that the disease can involve many parts of the body such as the heart, lungs, kidneys, and brain. SLE symptoms can be mild or serious.

- **Discoid lupus erythematosus** mainly affects the skin. A red rash may appear, or the skin on the face, scalp, or elsewhere may change color.

- **Drug-induced lupus** is triggered by a few medicines. It's like SLE, but symptoms are usually milder. Most of the time, the disease goes away when the medicine is stopped. More men develop drug-induced lupus because the drugs that cause it, hydralazine and procainamide, are used to treat heart conditions that are more common in men.

What Are The Signs And Symptoms Of Lupus?

Lupus may be hard to diagnose. It's often mistaken for other diseases. For this reason, lupus has been called the "great imitator." The signs of lupus differ from person to person. Some people have just a few signs; others have more.

Common signs of lupus are:

- Red rash or color change on the face, often in the shape of a butterfly across the nose and cheeks

- Painful or swollen joints

- Unexplained fever

- Chest pain with deep breathing

- Swollen glands

- Extreme fatigue (feeling tired all the time)

- Unusual hair loss (mainly on the scalp)

- Pale or purple fingers or toes from cold or stress

- Sensitivity to the sun

- Low blood count

- Depression, trouble thinking, and/or memory problems.

Other signs are mouth sores, unexplained seizures (convulsions), "seeing things" (hallucinations), repeated miscarriages, and unexplained kidney problems.

What Is A Flare?

When symptoms appear, it's called a "flare." These signs may come and go. You may have swelling and rashes one week and no symptoms at all the next. You may find that your symptoms flare after you've been out in the sun or after a hard day at work.

Even if you take medicine for lupus, you may find that there are times when the symptoms become worse. Learning to recognize that a flare is coming can help you take steps to cope with it. Many people feel very tired or have pain, a rash, a fever, stomach discomfort, headache, or dizziness just before a flare. Steps to prevent flares, such as limiting the time you spend in the sun (and artificial indoor light) and getting enough rest and quiet, can also be helpful.

Preventing A Flare
- Learn to recognize that a flare is coming.
- Talk with your doctor.
- Try to set realistic goals and priorities.
- Limit the time you spend in the sun (and artificial indoor light).
- Maintain a healthy diet.
- Develop coping skills to help limit stress.
- Get enough rest and quiet.
- Moderately exercise when possible.
- Develop a support system by surrounding yourself with people you trust and feel comfortable with (family, friends, etc.).

What Causes Lupus?

We don't know what causes lupus. There is no cure, but in most cases lupus can be managed. Lupus sometimes seems to run in families, which suggests the disease may be hereditary. Having the genes isn't the whole story, though. The environment, sunlight, stress, and certain medicines may trigger symptoms in some people. Other people who have similar genetic backgrounds may not get signs or symptoms of the disease. Researchers are trying to find out why.

Who Gets Lupus?

Anyone can get lupus. But we know that many more women than men get lupus. African American women are three times more likely to get lupus than white women. It's also more common in Hispanic/Latino, Asian, and American Indian women. Both African Americans and Hispanics/Latinos tend to develop lupus at a younger age and have more symptoms at diagnosis (including kidney problems).

They also tend to have more severe disease than whites. For example, African American patients have more seizures and strokes, while Hispanic/Latino patients have more heart problems. We don't understand why some people seem to have more problems with lupus than others.

Lupus is most common in women between the ages of 15 and 44. These are roughly the years when most women are able to have babies. Scientists think a woman's hormones may have something to do with getting lupus. But it's important to remember that men and older people can get it, too.

It's less common for children under age 15 to have lupus. One exception is babies born to women with lupus. These children may have heart, liver, or skin problems caused by lupus. With good care, most women with lupus can have a normal pregnancy and a healthy baby.

Diagnosis: How Do You Find Out If You Have Lupus?

- **Medical history.** Telling a doctor about your symptoms and other problems you have had can help him or her understand your situation. Your history can provide clues to your disease. Use the checklist at the end of this booklet to keep track of your symptoms. Share this checklist with your doctor. Ask your family or friends to help you with the checklist or come up with questions for your doctor.

- **Complete physical exam.** The doctor will look for rashes and other signs that something is wrong.

- **Laboratory testing of blood and urine samples.** Blood and urine samples often show if your immune system is overactive.

- **Skin or kidney biopsy.** In a biopsy, tissue that is removed by a minor surgical procedure is examined under a microscope. Skin or kidney tissue examined in this way can show signs of an autoimmune disease.

What Will The Doctor Do?

Go see a doctor. He or she will talk to you and take a history of your health problems. Many people have lupus for a long time before they find out they have it. It's important that you tell the doctor or nurse about your symptoms. This information, along with a physical examination and the results of laboratory tests, helps the doctor decide whether you have lupus or something else.

A rheumatologist is a doctor who specializes in treating diseases that affect the joints and muscles, like lupus. You may want to ask your regular doctor for a referral to a rheumatologist. In some cases, a dermatologist, a doctor who specializes in treating diseases that affect the skin, may be involved in diagnosis and treatment. No single test can show that you have lupus. Your doctor may have to run several tests and study your medical history. It may take time for the doctor to diagnose lupus.

Will I Get Medicine?

Remember that each person has different symptoms. Treatment depends on the symptoms. The doctor may give you aspirin or a similar medicine to treat swollen joints and fever. Creams may be prescribed for a rash. For more serious problems, stronger medicines such as antimalarial drugs, corticosteroids, chemotherapy drugs, and biologic drugs, including a B-lymphocyte stimulator (BLyS)-specific inhibitor, are used. Your doctor will choose a treatment based on your symptoms and needs.

Always tell your doctor if you have problems with your medicines. Let your doctor know if you take herbal or vitamin supplements. Your medicines may not mix well with these supplements. You and your doctor can work together to find the best way to treat all of your symptoms.

How Can I Cope With Lupus?

You need to find out what works best for you. You may find that a rheumatologist has the best treatment plan for you. Other health professionals who can help you deal with different aspects of lupus include psychologists, occupational therapists, dermatologists, and dietitians. You might find that doing exercises with a physical therapist makes you feel better. The important thing is to follow up with your healthcare team on a regular basis, even when your lupus is quiet and all seems well.

Dealing with a long-lasting disease like lupus can be hard on the emotions. You might think that your friends, family, and coworkers do not understand how you feel. Sadness and anger are common reactions.

People with lupus have limited energy and must manage it wisely. Ask your healthcare team about ways to cope with fatigue. Most people feel better if they manage their rest and work and take their medicine. If you're depressed, medicine and counseling can help.

Also,

- Pay attention to your body. Slow down or stop before you're too tired.

- Learn to pace yourself. Spread out your work and other activities.

- Don't blame yourself for your fatigue. It's part of the disease.

- Consider support groups and counseling. They can help you realize that you're not alone. Group members teach one another how to cope.

- Consider other support from your family as well as faith-based and other community groups.

It's true that staying healthy is harder when you have lupus. You need to pay close attention to your body, mind, and spirit. Having a chronic disease is stressful. People cope with stress differently. Some approaches that may help are:

- Staying involved in social activities.

- Practicing techniques such as meditation and yoga.

- Setting priorities for spending time and energy.

Exercising is another approach that can help you cope with lupus. Types of exercise that you can practice include the following:

- **Range-of-motion** (for example, stretching) exercise helps maintain normal joint movement and relieve stiffness. This type of exercise helps maintain or increase flexibility.

- **Strengthening** (for example, weight-lifting) exercises help keep or increase muscle strength. Strong muscles help support and protect joints affected by lupus.

- **Aerobic or endurance** (for example, brisk walking or jogging) exercises improve cardio-vascular fitness, help control weight, and improve overall function.

People with chronic diseases like lupus should check with their healthcare professional before starting an exercise program.

Learning about lupus may also help. People who are well-informed and take part in planning their own care, report less pain. They also may make fewer visits to the doctor, have more self-confidence, and remain more active.

Women who want to start a family should work closely with their healthcare team; for example, doctors, physical therapists, and nurses. Your obstetrician and your lupus doctor should work together to find the best treatment plan for you.

Chapter 38

Peptic Ulcers

A peptic ulcer is a sore in the lining of your stomach or your duodenum, the first part of your small intestine. A burning stomach pain is the most common symptom. The pain:

- Starts between meals or during the night

- Briefly stops if you eat or take antacids

- Lasts for minutes to hours

- Comes and goes for several days or weeks

Peptic ulcers happen when the acids that help you digest food damage the walls of the stomach or duodenum. The most common cause is infection with a bacterium called *Helicobacter pylori (H. pylori)*. Another cause is the long-term use of nonsteroidal anti-inflammatory medicines (NSAIDs) such as aspirin and ibuprofen. Stress and spicy foods do not cause ulcers, but can make them worse.

To see if you have an *H. pylori* infection, your doctor will test your blood, breath, or stool. Your doctor also may look inside your stomach and duodenum by doing an endoscopy or X-ray.

Peptic ulcers will get worse if not treated. Treatment may include medicines to reduce stomach acids or antibiotics to kill *H. pylori*. Antacids and milk can't heal peptic ulcers. Not smoking and avoiding alcohol can help. You may need surgery if your ulcers don't heal.

About This Chapter: Text in this chapter begins with excerpts from "Peptic Ulcer," MedlinePlus, National Institutes of Health (NIH), May 20, 2016; Text beginning with the heading "Symptoms And Causes Of Peptic Ulcers (Stomach Ulcers)" is excerpted from "Peptic Ulcers (Stomach Ulcers)," National Institute of Diabetes and Digestive and Kidney Diseases (NIDDK), November 2014. Reviewed October 2017.

What Are The Symptoms Of A Peptic Ulcer?

A dull or burning pain in your stomach is the most common symptom of a peptic ulcer. You may feel the pain anywhere between your belly button and breastbone. The pain most often:

- happens when your stomach is empty—such as between meals or during the night
- stops briefly if you eat or if you take antacids
- lasts for minutes to hours
- comes and goes for several days, weeks, or months

Less common symptoms may include:

- bloating
- burping
- feeling sick to your stomach
- poor appetite
- vomiting
- weight loss

Even if your symptoms are mild, you may have a peptic ulcer. You should see your doctor to talk about your symptoms. Without treatment, your peptic ulcer can get worse.

What Causes A Peptic Ulcer?

Causes of peptic ulcers include:

- long-term use of nonsteroidal anti-inflammatory drugs (NSAIDs), such as aspirin and ibuprofen
- an infection with the bacteria *Helicobacter pylori (H. pylori)*
- rare cancerous and noncancerous tumors in the stomach, duodenum, or pancreas—known as Zollinger-Ellison syndrome (ZES)

Sometimes peptic ulcers are caused by both NSAIDs and *H. pylori*.

How Do NSAIDs Cause A Peptic Ulcer?

To understand how NSAIDs cause peptic ulcer disease, it is important to understand how NSAIDs work. Nonsteroidal anti-inflammatory drugs reduce pain, fever, and inflammation, or swelling.

Everyone has two enzymes that produce chemicals in your body's cells that promote pain, inflammation, and fever. NSAIDs work by blocking or reducing the amount of these enzymes that your body makes. However, one of the enzymes also produces another type of chemical that protects the stomach lining from stomach acid and helps control bleeding. When NSAIDs block or reduce the amount of this enzyme in your body, they also increase your chance of developing a peptic ulcer.

How Do *H. Pylori* Cause A Peptic Ulcer And Peptic Ulcer Disease?

H. pylori are spiral-shaped bacteria that can cause peptic ulcer disease by damaging the mucous coating that protects the lining of the stomach and duodenum. Once *H. pylori* have damaged the mucous coating, powerful stomach acid can get through to the sensitive lining. Together, the stomach acid and *H. pylori* irritate the lining of the stomach or duodenum and cause a peptic ulcer.

How Do Tumors From ZES Cause Peptic Ulcers?

Zollinger-Ellison syndrome is a rare disorder that happens when one or more tumors form in your pancreas and duodenum. The tumors release large amounts of gastrin, a hormone that causes your stomach to produce large amounts of acid. The extra acid causes peptic ulcers to form in your duodenum and in the upper intestine.

How Do Doctors Diagnose A Peptic Ulcer?

Your doctor will use information from your medical history, a physical exam, and tests to diagnose an ulcer and its cause. The presence of an ulcer can only be determined by looking directly at the stomach with endoscopy or an X-ray test.

Medical History

To help diagnose a peptic ulcer, your doctor will ask you questions about your medical history, your symptoms, and the medicines you take.

Be sure to mention medicines that you take without a prescription, especially nonsteroidal anti-inflammatory drugs (NSAIDs), such as:

- aspirin (Bayer Aspirin)

- ibuprofen (Motrin, Advil)

- naproxen (Aleve)

Physical Exam

A physical exam may help a doctor diagnose a peptic ulcer. During a physical exam, a doctor most often:

- checks for bloating in your abdomen
- listens to sounds within your abdomen using a stethoscope
- taps on your abdomen checking for tenderness or pain

Lab Tests

To see if you have a *Helicobacter pylori (H. pylori)* infection, your doctor will order these tests:

Blood test: A blood test involves drawing a sample of your blood at your doctor's office or a commercial facility. A healthcare professional tests the blood sample to see if the results fall within the normal range for different disorders or infections.

Urea breath test: For a urea breath test, you will drink a special liquid that contains urea, a waste product that your body makes as it breaks down protein. If *H. pylori* are present, the bacteria will change this waste product into carbon dioxide—a harmless gas. Carbon dioxide normally appears in your breath when you exhale.

A healthcare professional will take a sample of your breath by having you breathe into a bag at your doctor's office or at a lab. He or she then sends your breath sample to a lab for testing. If your breath sample has higher levels of carbon dioxide than normal, you have *H. pylori* in your stomach or small intestine.

Stool test: Doctors use a stool test to study a sample of your stool. A doctor will give you a container for catching and storing your stool at home. You return the sample to the doctor or a commercial facility, who then sends it to a lab for analysis. Stool tests can show the presence of *H. pylori*.

Upper Gastrointestinal (GI) Endoscopy And Biopsy

In an upper GI endoscopy, a gastroenterologist, surgeon, or other trained healthcare professional uses an endoscope to see inside your upper GI tract. This procedure takes place at a hospital or an outpatient center.

An intravenous (IV) needle will be placed in your arm to provide a sedative. Sedatives help you stay relaxed and comfortable during the procedure. In some cases, the procedure can be performed without sedation. You will be given a liquid anesthetic to gargle or spray anesthetic on the back of your throat. The doctor will carefully feed the endoscope down your esophagus and into your stomach and duodenum. A small camera mounted on the endoscope sends a video image to a monitor, allowing close examination of the lining of your upper GI tract. The endoscope pumps air into your stomach and duodenum, making them easier to see.

The doctor may perform a biopsy with the endoscope by taking a small piece of tissue from the lining of your esophagus. You won't feel the biopsy. A pathologist examines the tissue in a lab.

Upper GI Series

An upper GI series looks at the shape of your upper GI tract. An X-ray technician performs this test at a hospital or an outpatient center. A radiologist reads and reports on the X-ray images. You don't need anesthesia. A healthcare professional will tell you how to prepare for the procedure, including when to stop eating and drinking.

During the procedure, you'll stand or sit in front of an X-ray machine and drink barium, a chalky liquid. Barium coats your esophagus, stomach, and small intestine so your doctor can see the shapes of these organs more clearly on X-rays.

You may have bloating and nausea for a short time after the test. For several days afterward, you may have white or light-colored stools from the barium. A healthcare professional will give you instructions about eating and drinking after the test.

Computerized Tomography (CT) Scan

A CT scan uses a combination of X-rays and computer technology to create images. For a CT scan, a healthcare professional may give you a solution to drink and an injection of a special dye, which doctors call contrast medium. You'll lie on a table that slides into a tunnel-shaped device that takes the X-rays. An X-ray technician performs the procedure in an outpatient center or a hospital, and a radiologist interprets the images. You don't need anesthesia.

CT scans can help diagnose a peptic ulcer that has created a hole in the wall of your stomach or small intestine.

How Do Doctors Treat Peptic Ulcer Disease?

There are several types of medicines used to treat a peptic ulcer. Your doctor will decide the best treatment based on the cause of your peptic ulcer.

How Do Doctors Treat An NSAID-Induced Peptic Ulcer?

If NSAIDs are causing your peptic ulcer and you don't have an *H. pylori* infection, your doctor may tell you to:

- stop taking the NSAID

- reduce how much of the NSAID you take

- switch to another medicine that won't cause a peptic ulcer

Your doctor may also prescribe medicines to reduce stomach acid and coat and protect your peptic ulcer. Proton pump inhibitors (PPIs), histamine receptor blockers, and protectants can help relieve pain and help your ulcer heal.

Proton Pump Inhibitor

PPIs reduce stomach acid and protect the lining of your stomach and duodenum. While PPIs can't kill *H. pylori*, they do help fight the *H. pylori* infection.

PPIs include:

- esomeprazole (Nexium)

- dexlansoprazole (Dexilant)

- lansoprazole (Prevacid)

- omeprazole (Prilosec, Zegerid)

- pantoprazole (Protonix)

- rabeprazole (AcipHex)

Histamine Receptor Blockers

Histamine receptor blockers work by blocking histamine, a chemical in your body that signals your stomach to produce acid. Histamine receptor blockers include:

- cimetidine (Tagamet)

- famotidine (Pepcid)

- ranitidine (Zantac)

- nizatidine (Axid) Protectants

Protectants

Protectants coat ulcers and protect them against acid and enzymes so that healing can occur. Doctors only prescribe one—sucralfate (Carafate)—for peptic ulcer disease. Tell your doctor if the medicines make you feel sick or dizzy or cause diarrhea or headaches. Your doctor can change your medicines.

If you smoke, quit. You also should avoid alcohol. Drinking alcohol and smoking slow the healing of a peptic ulcer and can make it worse.

What If I Still Need To Take NSAIDS?

If you take NSAIDs for other conditions, such as arthritis, you should talk with your doctor about the benefits and risks of using NSAIDs. Your doctor can help you determine how to continue using an NSAID safely after your peptic ulcer symptoms go away. Your doctor may prescribe a medicine used to prevent NSAID-induced ulcers called Misoprosotol.

Tell your doctor about all the prescription and over-the-counter medicines you take. Your doctor can then decide if you may safely take NSAIDs or if you should switch to a different medicine. In either case, your doctor may prescribe a PPI or histamine receptor blocker to protect the lining of your stomach and duodenum.

If you need NSAIDs, you can reduce the chance of a peptic ulcer returning by:

- taking the NSAID with a meal
- using the lowest effective dose possible
- quitting smoking
- avoiding alcohol

How Do Doctors Treat An NSAID-Induced Peptic Ulcer When You Have An *H. Pylori* Infection?

If you have an *H. pylori* infection, a doctor will treat your NSAID-induced peptic ulcer with PPIs or histamine receptor blockers and other medicines, such as antibiotics, bismuth subsalicylates, or antacids.

PPIs reduce stomach acid and protect the lining of your stomach and duodenum. While PPIs can't kill *H. pylori,* they do help fight the *H. pylori* infection.

PPIs include:

- esomeprazole (Nexium)
- dexlansoprazole (Dexilant)
- lansoprazole (Prevacid)

- omeprazole (Prilosec, Zegerid)
- pantoprazole (Protonix)
- rabeprazole (AcipHex)

Histamine Receptor Blockers

Histamine receptor blockers work by blocking histamine, a chemical in your body that signals your stomach to produce acid. Histamine receptor blockers include:

- cimetidine (Tagamet)
- famotidine (Pepcid)
- ranitidine (Zantac)
- nizatidine (Axid)

Antibiotics

A doctor will prescribe antibiotics to kill *H. pylori*. How doctors prescribe antibiotics may differ throughout the world. Over time, some types of antibiotics can no longer destroy certain types of *H. pylori*.

Antibiotics can cure most peptic ulcers caused by *H. pylori or H. pylori*-induced peptic ulcers. However, getting rid of the bacteria can be difficult. Take all doses of your antibiotics exactly as your doctor prescribes, even if the pain from a peptic ulcer is gone.

Bismuth Subsalicylates

Medicines containing bismuth subsalicylate, such as Pepto-Bismol, coat a peptic ulcer and protect it from stomach acid. Although bismuth subsalicylate can kill *H. pylori,* doctors sometimes prescribe it with antibiotics, not in place of antibiotics.

Antacids

An antacid may make the pain from a peptic ulcer go away temporarily, yet it will not kill *H. pylori*. If you receive treatment for an *H. pylori*-induced peptic ulcer, check with your doctor before taking antacids. Some of the antibiotics may not work as well if you take them with an antacid.

How Do Doctors Treat An *H. pylori*-Induced Peptic Ulcer?

Doctors may prescribe triple therapy, quadruple therapy, or sequential therapy to treat an *H. pylori*-induced peptic ulcer.

Triple Therapy

For triple therapy, your doctor will prescribe that you take the following for 7 to 14 days:

- the antibiotic clarithromycin
- the antibiotic metronidazole or the antibiotic amoxicillin
- a PPI

Quadruple Therapy

For quadruple therapy, your doctor will prescribe that you take the following for 14 days:

- a PPI
- bismuth subsalicylate
- the antibiotics tetracycline and metronidazole

Doctors prescribe quadruple therapy to treat patients who:

- can't take amoxicillin because of an allergy to penicillin. Penicillin and amoxicillin are similar.
- have previously received a macrolide antibiotic, such as clarithromycin.
- are still infected with *H. pylori* after triple therapy treatment.

Doctors prescribe quadruple therapy after the first treatment has failed. In the second round of treatment, the doctor may prescribe different antibiotics than those that he or she prescribed the first time.

Sequential Therapy

For sequential therapy, your doctor will prescribe that you take the following for 5 days:

- a PPI
- amoxicillin

Then the doctor will prescribe you the following for another 5 days:

- a PPI
- clarithromycin
- the antibiotic tinidazole

Triple therapy, quadruple therapy, and sequential therapy may cause nausea and other side effects, including:

- an altered sense of taste

- darkened stools

- a darkened tongue

- diarrhea

- headaches

- temporary reddening of the skin when drinking alcohol

- vaginal yeast infections

Talk with your doctor about any side effects that bother you. He or she may prescribe you other medicines.

How Do Doctors Treat Peptic Ulcers Caused By ZES?

Doctors use medicines, surgery, and chemotherapy to treat Zollinger-Ellison syndrome. Learn more about Zollinger-Ellison syndrome treatment.

What If A Peptic Ulcer Doesn't Heal?

Most often, medicines heal a peptic ulcer. If an *H. pylori* infection caused your peptic ulcer, you should finish all of your antibiotics and take any other medicines your doctor prescribes. The infection and peptic ulcer will heal only if you take all medicines as your doctor prescribes.

When you have finished your medicines, your doctor may do another breath or stool test in 4 weeks or more to be sure the *H. pylori* infection is gone. Sometimes, *H. pylori* bacteria are still present, even after you have taken all the medicines correctly. If the infection is still present, your peptic ulcer could return or, rarely, stomach cancer could develop. Your doctor will prescribe different antibiotics to get rid of the infection and cure your peptic ulcer.

Can A Peptic Ulcer Come Back?

Yes, a peptic ulcer can come back. If you smoke or take NSAIDs, peptic ulcers are more likely to come back. If you need to take an NSAID, your doctor may switch you to a different medicine or add medicines to help prevent a peptic ulcer. Peptic ulcer disease can return, even if you have been careful to reduce your risk.

How Can I Prevent A Peptic Ulcer?

To help prevent a peptic ulcer caused by NSAIDs, ask your doctor if you should:

- stop using NSAIDs

- take NSAIDs with a meal if you still need NSAIDs

- take a lower dose of NSAIDs

- take medicines to protect your stomach and duodenum while taking NSAIDs

- switch to a medicine that won't cause ulcers

To help prevent a peptic ulcer caused by *H. pylori,* your doctor may recommend that you avoid drinking alcohol.

How Can Your Diet Help Prevent Or Relieve A Peptic Ulcer?

Researchers have not found that diet and nutrition play an important role in causing or preventing peptic ulcers. Before acid blocking drugs became available, milk was used to treat ulcers. However, milk is not an effective way to prevent or relieve a peptic ulcer. Alcohol and smoking do contribute to ulcers and should be avoided.

Chapter 39

Acid Reflux (GER And GERD)

What Is GER?

Gastroesophageal reflux (GER) happens when stomach contents come back up into the esophagus. Stomach acid that touches the lining of the esophagus can cause heartburn, also called acid indigestion.

Does GER Have Another Name?

Doctors also refer to GER as:

- acid indigestion
- acid reflux
- acid regurgitation
- heartburn
- reflux

How Common Is GER In Children And Teens?

Occasional GER is common in children and teens—ages 2 to 19—and doesn't always mean that they have gastroesophageal reflux disease (GERD).

About This Chapter: This chapter includes text excerpted from "Acid Reflux (GER And GERD) In Children And Teens," National Institute of Diabetes and Digestive and Kidney Diseases (NIDDK), April 2015.

What Is GERD?

Gastroesophageal Reflux Disease (GERD) is a more serious and long-lasting form of GER in which acid reflux irritates the esophagus.

What Is The Difference Between GER And GERD?

GER that occurs more than twice a week for a few weeks could be GERD. GERD can lead to more serious health problems over time. If you think your child or teen has GERD, you should take him or her to see a doctor or a pediatrician.

How Common Is GERD In Children And Teens?

Up to 25 percent of children and teens have symptoms of GERD, although GERD is more common in adults.

What Are The Complications Of GERD In Children And Teens?

Without treatment, GERD can sometimes cause serious complications over time, such as:

Esophagitis

Esophagitis may lead to ulcerations, a sore in the lining of the esophagus.

Esophageal Stricture

An esophageal stricture happens when a person's esophagus becomes too narrow. Esophageal strictures can lead to problems with swallowing.

Respiratory Problems

A child or teen with GERD might breathe stomach acid into his or her lungs. The stomach acid can then irritate his or her throat and lungs, causing respiratory problems or symptoms, such as

- asthma—a long-lasting lung disease that makes a child or teen extra sensitive to things that he or she is allergic to

- chest congestion, or extra fluid in the lungs

- a dry, long-lasting cough or a sore throat

- hoarseness—the partial loss of a child or teen's voice
- laryngitis—the swelling of a child or teen's voice box that can lead to a short-term loss of his or her voice
- pneumonia—an infection in one or both lungs—that keeps coming back
- wheezing—a high-pitched whistling sound that happens while breathing

A pediatrician should monitor children and teens with GERD to prevent or treat long-term problems.

What Are The Symptoms Of GER And GERD In Children And Teens?

If a child or teen has gastroesophageal reflux (GER), he or she may taste food or stomach acid in the back of the mouth.

Symptoms of gastroesophageal reflux disease (GERD) in children and teens can vary depending on their age. The most common symptom of GERD in children 12 years and older is regular heartburn, a painful, burning feeling in the middle of the chest, behind the breast-bone, and in the middle of the abdomen. In many cases, children with GERD who are younger than 12 don't have heartburn.

Other common GERD symptoms include

- bad breath
- nausea
- pain in the chest or the upper part of the abdomen
- problems swallowing or painful swallowing
- respiratory problems
- vomiting
- the wearing away of teeth

What Causes GER And GERD In Children And Teens?

GER and GERD happen when a child or teen's lower esophageal sphincter becomes weak or relaxes when it shouldn't, causing stomach contents to rise up into the esophagus. The lower esophageal sphincter becomes weak or relaxes due to certain things, such as:

- increased pressure on the abdomen from being overweight, obese, or pregnant

- certain medicines, including:

  - those used to treat asthma—a long-lasting disease in the lungs that makes a child or teen extra sensitive to things that he or she is allergic to

  - antihistamines—medicines that treat allergy symptoms

  - painkillers

  - sedatives—medicines that help put someone to sleep

  - antidepressants—medicines that treat depression

- Smoking, which is more likely with teens than younger children, or inhaling second-hand smoke

Other reasons a child or teen develops GERD include:

- previous esophageal surgery

- having a severe developmental delay or neurological condition, such as cerebral palsy

When Should I Seek A Doctor's Help?

Call a doctor right away if your child or teen vomits large amounts has regular projectile, or forceful, vomiting

- vomits fluid that is

  - green or yellow

  - looks like coffee grounds

  - contains blood

- has problems breathing after vomiting

- has mouth of throat pain when he or she eats

- has problems swallowing or pain when swallowing

- refuses food repeatedly, causing weight loss or poor growth

- shows signs of dehydration, such as no tears when he or she cries

How Do Doctors Diagnose GERD In Children And Teens?

In most cases, a doctor diagnoses gastroesophageal reflux (GER) by reviewing a child or teen's symptoms and medical history. If symptoms of GER do not improve with lifestyle changes and antireflux medicines, he or she may need testing.

How Do Doctors Treat GER And GERD In Children And Teens?

If a child or teen's GER symptoms do not improve, if they come back frequently, or he or she has trouble swallowing, the doctor may recommend testing for gastroesophageal reflux disease (GERD).

The doctor may refer the child or teen to a pediatric gastroenterologist to diagnose and treat GERD.

How Do Doctors Treat GERD In Children And Teens?

You can help control a child or teen's gastroesophageal reflux (GER) or gastroesophageal reflux disease (GERD) by having him or her

- not eat or drink items that may cause GER, such as greasy or spicy foods

- not overeat

- avoid smoking and secondhand smoke

- lose weight if he or she is overweight or obese

- avoid eating 2 to 3 hours before bedtime

- take over-the-counter medicines, such as Alka-Seltzer, Maalox, or Rolaids

How Can Diet Help Prevent Or Relieve GER Or GERD In Children And Teens?

Depending on the severity of the child's symptoms, a doctor may recommend lifestyle changes, medicines, or surgery.

Lifestyle Changes

Helping a child or teen make lifestyle changes can reduce his or her GERD symptoms. A child or teen should

- lose weight, if needed.

- eat smaller meals

- avoid high-fat foods

- wear loose-fitting clothing around the abdomen. Tight clothing can squeeze the stomach area and push the acid up into the esophagus.

- stay upright for 3 hours after meals and avoid reclining and slouching when sitting.

- sleep at a slight angle. Raise the head of the child or teen's bed 6 to 8 inches by safely putting blocks under the bedposts. Just using extra pillows will not help.

- If a teen smokes, help them quit smoking and avoid secondhand smoke.

Over-The-Counter And Prescription Medicines

If a child or teen has symptoms that won't go away, you should take him or her to see a doctor. The doctor can prescribe medicine to relieve his or her symptoms. Some medicines are available over the counter.

All GERD medicines work in different ways. A child or teen may need a combination of GERD medicines to control symptoms.

Antacids

Doctors often first recommend antacids to relieve GER and other mild GERD symptoms. A doctor will tell you which over-the-counter antacids to give a child or teen, such as

- Alka-Seltzer

- Maalox

- Mylanta

- Riopan

- Rolaids

Antacids can have side effects, including diarrhea and constipation. Don't give your child or teen over-the-counter antacids without first checking with his or her doctor.

H2 Blockers

H2 blockers decrease acid production. They provide short-term or on-demand relief for many people with GERD symptoms. They can also help heal the esophagus, although not as well as other medicines. If a doctor recommends an H2 blocker for the child or teen, you can buy them over the counter or a doctor can prescribe one. Types of H2 blockers include

- cimetidine (Tagamet HB)

- famotidine (Pepcid AC)

- nizatidine (Axid AR)

- ranitidine (Zantac 75)

If a child or teen develops heartburn after eating, his or her doctor may prescribe an antacid and an H2 blocker. The antacids neutralize stomach acid, and the H2 blockers stop the stomach from creating acid. By the time the antacids wear off, the H2 blockers are controlling the acid in the stomach.

Don't give your child or teen over-the-counter H2 blockers without first checking with his or her doctor.

Proton Pump Inhibitors (PPIs)

PPIs lower the amount of acid the stomach makes. PPIs are better at treating GERD symptoms than H2 blockers. They can heal the esophageal lining in most people with GERD. Doctors often prescribe PPIs for long-term GERD treatment.

However, studies show that people who take PPIs for a long time or in high doses are more likely to have hip, wrist, and spinal fractures. A child or teen should take these medicines on an empty stomach so that his or her stomach acid can make them work correctly.

Several types of PPIs are available by a doctor's prescription, including

- esomeprazole (Nexium)

- lansoprazole (Prevacid)

- omeprazole (Prilosec, Zegerid)

- pantoprazole (Protonix)

- rabeprazole (AcipHex)

Talk with the child or teen's doctor about taking lower-strength omeprazole or lansoprazole, sold over the counter. Don't give a child or teen over-the-counter PPIs without first checking with his or her doctor.

Prokinetics

Prokinetics help the stomach empty faster. Prescription prokinetics include

- bethanechol (Urecholine)

- metoclopramide (Reglan)

Both these medicines have side effects, including

- nausea

- diarrhea

- fatigue, or feeling tired

- depression

- anxiety

- delayed or abnormal physical movement

Prokinetics can cause problems if a child or teen mixes them with other medicines, so tell the doctor about all the medicines he or she is taking.

Antibiotics

Antibiotics, including erythromycin, can help the stomach empty faster. Erythromycin has fewer side effects than prokinetics; however, it can cause diarrhea.

Surgery

A pediatric gastroenterologist may recommend surgery if a child or teen's GERD symptoms don't improve with lifestyle changes or medicines. A child or teen is more likely to develop complications from surgery than from medicines.

Fundoplication is the most common surgery for GERD. In most cases, it leads to long-term reflux control.

A surgeon performs fundoplication using a laparoscope, a thin tube with a tiny video camera. During the operation, a surgeon sews the top of the stomach around the esophagus to add pressure to the lower end of the esophagus and reduce reflux.

The surgeon performs the operation at a hospital. The child or teen receives general anesthesia and can leave the hospital in 1 to 3 days. Most children and teens return to their usual daily activities in 2 to 3 weeks.

Endoscopic techniques, such as endoscopic sewing and radiofrequency, help control GERD in a small number of people. Endoscopic sewing uses small stitches to tighten the sphincter muscle. Radiofrequency creates heat lesions, or sores, that help tighten the sphincter muscle. A surgeon performs both operations using an endoscope at a hospital or an outpatient center, and the child or teen receives general anesthesia.

The results for endoscopic techniques may not be as good as those for fundoplication. Doctors don't use endoscopic techniques.

What Should A Child Or Teen With GERD Avoid Eating Or Drinking?

You can help a child or teen prevent or relieve their symptoms from gastroesophageal reflux (GER) or gastroesophageal reflux disease (GERD) by changing their diet. He or she may need to avoid certain foods and drinks that make his or her symptoms worse. Other dietary changes that can help reduce the child or teen's symptoms include

- decreasing fatty foods
- eating small, frequent meals instead of three large meals

What Can A Child Or Teen Eat If They Have GERD?

He or she should avoid eating or drinking the following items that may make GER or GERD worse

- chocolate
- coffee
- peppermint
- greasy or spicy foods
- tomatoes and tomato products

How Do Doctors Diagnose GER In Children And Teens?

Eating healthy and balanced amounts of different types of foods is good for your child or teen's overall health. If your child or teen is overweight or obese, talk with a doctor or dietitian about dietary changes that can help with losing weight and decreasing the GERD symptoms.

Chapter 40

Irritable Bowel Syndrome (IBS)

What Is Irritable Bowel Syndrome (IBS)?

Irritable bowel syndrome is a functional gastrointestinal (GI) disorder, meaning it is a problem caused by changes in how the GI tract works. Children with a functional GI disorder have frequent symptoms, but the GI tract does not become damaged. IBS is not a disease; it is a group of symptoms that occur together. The most common symptoms of IBS are abdominal pain or discomfort, often reported as cramping, along with diarrhea, constipation, or both. In the past, IBS was called colitis, mucous colitis, spastic colon, nervous colon, and spastic bowel. The name was changed to reflect the understanding that the disorder has both physical and mental causes and is not a product of a person's imagination.

IBS is diagnosed when a child who is growing as expected has abdominal pain or discomfort once per week for at least 2 months without other disease or injury that could explain the pain. The pain or discomfort of IBS may occur with a change in stool frequency or consistency or may be relieved by a bowel movement.

What Is The GI Tract?

The GI tract is a series of hollow organs joined in a long, twisting tube from the mouth to the anus. The movement of muscles in the GI tract, along with the release of hormones and enzymes, allows for the digestion of food. Organs that make up the GI tract are the

About This Chapter: This chapter includes text excerpted from "Irritable Bowel Syndrome (IBS) In Children," National Institute of Diabetes and Digestive and Kidney Diseases (NIDDK), June 2014. Reviewed October 2017.

mouth, esophagus, stomach, small intestine, large intestine—which includes the appendix, cecum, colon, and rectum—and anus. The intestines are sometimes called the bowel. The last part of the GI tract—called the lower GI tract—consists of the large intestine and anus.

The large intestine absorbs water and any remaining nutrients from partially digested food passed from the small intestine. The large intestine then changes waste from liquid to a solid matter called stool. Stool passes from the colon to the rectum. The rectum is located between the last parts of the colon—called the sigmoid colon—and the anus. The rectum stores stool prior to a bowel movement. During a bowel movement, stool moves from the rectum to the anus, the opening through which stool leaves the body.

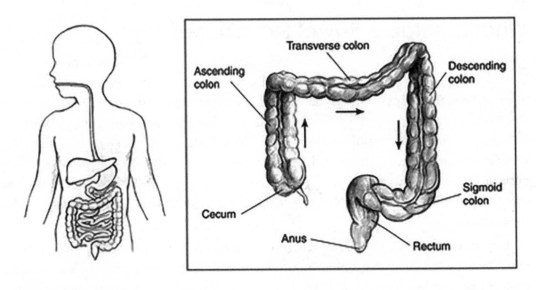

Figure 40.1. The Lower GI Tract

How Common Is IBS In Children?

Limited information is available about the number of children with IBS. Older studies have reported prevalence rates for recurrent abdominal pain in children of 10 to 20 percent. However, these studies did not differentiate IBS from functional abdominal pain, indigestion, and abdominal migraine. One study of children in North America found that 14 percent of high school students and 6 percent of middle school students have IBS. The study also found that IBS affects boys and girls equally.

What Are The Symptoms Of IBS In Children?

The symptoms of IBS include abdominal pain or discomfort and changes in bowel habits. To meet the definition of IBS, the pain or discomfort should be associated with two of the following three symptoms:

- start with bowel movements that occur more or less often than usual
- start with stool that appears looser and more watery or harder and more lumpy than usual
- improve with a bowel movement

Other symptoms of IBS may include:

- diarrhea—having loose, watery stools three or more times a day and feeling urgency to have a bowel movement
- constipation—having hard, dry stools; two or fewer bowel movements in a week; or straining to have a bowel movement
- feeling that a bowel movement is incomplete
- passing mucus, a clear liquid made by the intestines that coats and protects tissues in the GI tract
- abdominal bloating

Symptoms may often occur after eating a meal. To meet the definition of IBS, symptoms must occur at least once per week for at least 2 months.

What Causes IBS In Children?

The causes of IBS are not well understood. Researchers believe a combination of physical and mental health problems can lead to IBS. The possible causes of IBS in children include the following:

- **Brain-gut signal problems.** Signals between the brain and nerves of the small and large intestines, also called the gut, control how the intestines work. Problems with brain-gut signals may cause IBS symptoms, such as changes in bowel habits and pain or discomfort.

- **GI motor problems.** Normal motility, or movement, may not be present in the colon of a child who has IBS. Slow motility can lead to constipation and fast motility can lead to diarrhea. Spasms, or sudden strong muscle contractions that come and go, can cause abdominal pain. Some children with IBS also experience hyperreactivity, which is an excessive increase in contractions of the bowel in response to stress or eating.

- **Hypersensitivity.** Children with IBS have greater sensitivity to abdominal pain than children without IBS. Affected children have been found to have different rectal tone and rectal motor response after eating a meal.

- **Mental health problems.** IBS has been linked to mental health, or psychological, problems such as anxiety and depression in children.

- **Bacterial gastroenteritis.** Some children who have bacterial gastroenteritis—an infection or irritation of the stomach and intestines caused by bacteria—develop IBS. Research has shown a connection between gastroenteritis and IBS in adults but not in children. But researchers believe postinfectious IBS does occur in children. Researchers do not know why gastroenteritis leads to IBS in some people and not others.

- **Small intestinal bacterial overgrowth (SIBO).** Normally, few bacteria live in the small intestine. SIBO is an increase in the number of bacteria or a change in the type of bacteria in the small intestine. These bacteria can produce excess gas and may also cause diarrhea and weight loss. Some researchers believe that SIBO may lead to IBS, and some studies have shown antibiotics to be effective in treating IBS. However, the studies were weak and more research is needed to show a link between SIBO and IBS.

- **Genetics.** Whether IBS has a genetic cause, meaning it runs in families, is unclear. Studies have shown that IBS is more common in people with family members who have a history of GI problems. However, the cause could be environmental or the result of heightened awareness of GI symptoms.

How Is IBS In Children Diagnosed?

To diagnose IBS, a healthcare provider will conduct a physical exam and take a complete medical history. The medical history will include questions about the child's symptoms, family members with GI disorders, recent infections, medications, and stressful events related to the onset of symptoms. IBS is diagnosed when the physical exam does not show any cause for the child's symptoms and the child meets all of the following criteria:

- has had symptoms at least once per week for at least 2 months

- is growing as expected

- is not showing any signs that suggest another cause for the symptoms

Further testing is not usually needed, though the healthcare provider may do a blood test to screen for other problems. Additional diagnostic tests may be needed based on the results of the screening blood test and for children who also have signs such as:

- persistent pain in the upper right or lower right area of the abdomen

- joint pain

- pain that wakes them from sleep

- disease in the tissues around the rectum

- difficulty swallowing

- persistent vomiting

- slowed growth rate

- GI bleeding

- delayed puberty

- diarrhea at night

Further diagnostic tests may also be needed for children with a family history of:

- inflammatory bowel disease—long-lasting disorders that cause irritation and ulcers, or sores, in the GI tract

- celiac disease—an immune disease in which people cannot tolerate gluten, a protein found in wheat, rye, and barley, because it will damage the lining of their small intestine and prevent absorption of nutrients

- peptic ulcer disease—a sore in the lining of the esophagus or stomach

Additional diagnostic tests may include a stool test, ultrasound, and flexible sigmoidoscopy or colonoscopy.

Stool tests. A stool test is the analysis of a sample of stool. The healthcare provider will give the child's caretaker a container for catching and storing the child's stool. The sample is returned to the healthcare provider or a commercial facility and sent to a lab for analysis. The healthcare provider may also do a rectal exam, sometimes during the physical exam, to check for blood in the stool. Stool tests can show the presence of parasites or blood.

Ultrasound. Ultrasound uses a device, called a transducer, that bounces safe, painless sound waves off organs to create an image of their structure. The procedure is performed in a healthcare provider's office, outpatient center, or hospital by a specially trained technician, and the images are interpreted by a radiologist—a doctor who specializes in medical imaging; anesthesia is not needed. The images can show problems in the GI tract causing pain or other symptoms.

Flexible sigmoidoscopy or colonoscopy. The tests are similar, but a colonoscopy is used to view the rectum and entire colon, while a flexible sigmoidoscopy is used to view just the rectum and lower colon. These tests are performed at a hospital or outpatient center by a gastroenterologist—a doctor who specializes in digestive diseases. For both tests, a healthcare provider will give written bowel prep instructions to follow at home. The child may be asked to follow a clear liquid diet for 1 to 3 days before either test. The night before the test, the child may need to take a laxative. One or more enemas may also be required the night before and about 2 hours before the test.

In most cases, light anesthesia, and possibly pain medication, helps the child relax. For either test, the child will lie on a table while the gastroenterologist inserts a flexible tube into the anus. A small camera on the tube sends a video image of the intestinal lining to a computer screen. The test can show signs of problems in the lower GI tract.

The gastroenterologist may also perform a biopsy, a procedure that involves taking a piece of intestinal lining for examination with a microscope. The child will not feel the biopsy. A pathologist—a doctor who specializes in diagnosing diseases—examines the tissue in a lab.

Cramping or bloating may occur during the first hour after the test. Full recovery is expected by the next day.

How Is IBS In Children Treated?

Though there is no cure for IBS, the symptoms can be treated with a combination of the following:

- changes in eating, diet, and nutrition
- medications
- probiotics
- therapies for mental health problems

Eating, Diet, And Nutrition

Large meals can cause cramping and diarrhea, so eating smaller meals more often, or eating smaller portions, may help IBS symptoms. Eating meals that are low in fat and high in carbohydrates, such as pasta, rice, whole-grain breads and cereals, fruits, and vegetables may help.

Certain foods and drinks may cause IBS symptoms in some children, such as:

- foods high in fat

- milk products

- drinks with caffeine

- drinks with large amounts of artificial sweeteners, which are substances used in place of sugar

- foods that may cause gas, such as beans and cabbage

Children with IBS may want to limit or avoid these foods. Keeping a food diary is a good way to track which foods cause symptoms so they can be excluded from or reduced in the diet.

Dietary fiber may lessen constipation in children with IBS, but it may not help with lowering pain. Fiber helps keep stool soft so it moves smoothly through the colon. The Academy of Nutrition and Dietetics recommends children consume "age plus 5" grams of fiber daily. A 7-year-old child, for example, should get "7 plus 5," or 12 grams, of fiber a day.3 Fiber may cause gas and trigger symptoms in some children with IBS. Increasing fiber intake by 2 to 3 grams per day may help reduce the risk of increased gas and bloating.

Medications

The healthcare provider will select medications based on the child's symptoms. Caregivers should not give children any medications unless told to do so by a healthcare provider.

- **Fiber supplements.** Fiber supplements may be recommended to relieve constipation when increasing dietary fiber is ineffective.

- **Laxatives.** Constipation can be treated with laxative medications. Laxatives work in different ways, and a healthcare provider can provide information about which type is best. Caregivers should not give children laxatives unless told to do so by a healthcare provider.

- **Antidiarrheals.** Loperamide has been found to reduce diarrhea in children with IBS, though it does not reduce pain, bloating, or other symptoms. Loperamide reduces stool frequency and improves stool consistency by slowing the movement of stool through the colon. Medications to treat diarrhea in adults can be dangerous for infants and children and should only be given if told to do so by a healthcare provider.

- **Antispasmodics.** Antispasmodics, such as hyoscine, cimetropium, and pinaverium, help to control colon muscle spasms and reduce abdominal pain.

- **Antidepressants.** Tricyclic antidepressants and selective serotonin reuptake inhibitors in low doses can help relieve IBS symptoms including abdominal pain. These medications are thought to reduce the perception of pain, improve mood and sleep patterns, and adjust the activity of the GI tract.

Probiotics

Probiotics are live microorganisms, usually bacteria, that are similar to microorganisms normally found in the GI tract. Studies have found that probiotics, specifically *Bifidobacteria* and certain probiotic combinations, improve symptoms of IBS when taken in large enough amounts. But more research is needed. Probiotics can be found in dietary supplements, such as capsules, tablets, and powders, and in some foods, such as yogurt. A healthcare provider can give information about the right kind and right amount of probiotics to take to improve IBS symptoms.

Therapies For Mental Health Problems

The following therapies can help improve IBS symptoms due to mental health problems:

- **Talk therapy.** Talking with a therapist may reduce stress and improve IBS symptoms. Two types of talk therapy used to treat IBS are cognitive behavioral therapy and psychodynamic, or interpersonal, therapy. Cognitive behavioral therapy focuses on the child's thoughts and actions. Psychodynamic therapy focuses on how emotions affect IBS symptoms. This type of therapy often involves relaxation and stress management techniques.

- **Hypnotherapy.** In hypnotherapy, the therapist uses hypnosis to help the child relax into a trancelike state. This type of therapy may help the child relax the muscles in the colon.

Chapter 41

Ulcerative Colitis

Ulcerative colitis (UC) is a disease that causes inflammation and sores, called ulcers, in the lining of the rectum and colon. It is one of a group of diseases called inflammatory bowel disease. UC can happen at any age, but it usually starts between the ages of 15 and 30. It tends to run in families. The most common symptoms are pain in the abdomen and blood or pus in diarrhea. Other symptoms may include:

- Anemia

- Severe tiredness

- Weight loss

- Loss of appetite

- Bleeding from the rectum

- Sores on the skin

- Joint pain

- Growth failure in children

About half of people with UC have mild symptoms. Doctors use blood tests, stool tests, colonoscopy or sigmoidoscopy, and imaging tests to diagnose UC. Several types of drugs can help control it. Some people have long periods of remission, when they are free of symptoms. In severe cases, doctors must remove the colon.

About This Chapter: Text in this chapter begins with excerpts from "Ulcerative Colitis" MedlinePlus, National Institutes of Health (NIH), June 14, 2016; Text under the heading "What Is The Large Intestine?" is excerpted from "Ulcerative Colitis," National Institute of Diabetes and Digestive and Kidney Diseases (NIDDK), September 2014. Reviewed October 2017.

What Is The Large Intestine?

The large intestine is part of the GI tract, a series of hollow organs joined in a long, twisting tube from the mouth to the anus—an opening through which stool leaves the body. The last part of the GI tract, called the lower GI tract, consists of the large intestine—which includes the appendix, cecum, colon, and rectum—and anus. The intestines are sometimes called the bowel.

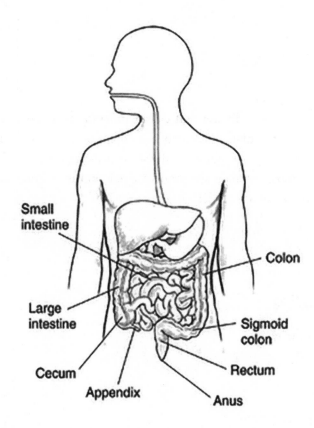

Figure 41.1. Large Intestine Is Part Of The GI Tract

The large intestine is about 5 feet long in adults and absorbs water and any remaining nutrients from partially digested food passed from the small intestine. The large intestine changes waste from liquid to a solid matter called stool. Stool passes from the colon to the rectum. The rectum is located between the lower, or sigmoid, colon and the anus. The rectum stores stool prior to a bowel movement, when stool moves from the rectum to the anus and out of a person's body.

What Causes Ulcerative Colitis?

The exact cause of ulcerative colitis is unknown. Researchers believe the following factors may play a role in causing ulcerative colitis:

- overactive intestinal immune system

- genes

- environment

Overactive intestinal immune system. Scientists believe one cause of ulcerative colitis may be an abnormal immune reaction in the intestine. Normally, the immune system protects the body from infection by identifying and destroying bacteria, viruses, and other potentially harmful foreign substances. Researchers believe bacteria or viruses can mistakenly trigger the immune system to attack the inner lining of the large intestine. This immune system response causes the inflammation, leading to symptoms.

Genes. Ulcerative colitis sometimes runs in families. Research studies have shown that certain abnormal genes may appear in people with ulcerative colitis. However, researchers have not been able to show a clear link between the abnormal genes and ulcerative colitis.

Environment. Some studies suggest that certain things in the environment may increase the chance of a person getting ulcerative colitis, although the overall chance is low. Nonsteroidal anti-inflammatory drugs, antibiotics, and oral contraceptives may slightly increase the chance of developing ulcerative colitis. A high-fat diet may also slightly increase the chance of getting ulcerative colitis.

Some people believe eating certain foods, stress, or emotional distress can cause ulcerative colitis. Emotional distress does not seem to cause ulcerative colitis. A few studies suggest that stress may increase a person's chance of having a flare-up of ulcerative colitis. Also, some people may find that certain foods can trigger or worsen symptoms.

Who Is More Likely To Develop Ulcerative Colitis?

Ulcerative colitis can occur in people of any age. However, it is more likely to develop in people

- between the ages of 15 and 30

- older than 60

- who have a family member with IBD
- of Jewish descent

What Are The Signs And Symptoms Of Ulcerative Colitis?

The most common signs and symptoms of ulcerative colitis are diarrhea with blood or pus and abdominal discomfort. Other signs and symptoms include:

- an urgent need to have a bowel movement
- feeling tired
- nausea or loss of appetite
- weight loss
- fever
- anemia—a condition in which the body has fewer red blood cells than normal

Less common symptoms include:

- joint pain or soreness
- eye irritation
- certain rashes

The symptoms a person experiences can vary depending on the severity of the inflammation and where it occurs in the intestine. When symptoms first appear,

- most people with ulcerative colitis have mild to moderate symptoms
- about 10 percent of people can have severe symptoms, such as frequent, bloody bowel movements; fevers; and severe abdominal cramping.

How Is Ulcerative Colitis Diagnosed?

A healthcare provider diagnoses ulcerative colitis with the following:

- medical and family history
- physical exam
- lab tests
- endoscopies of the large intestine

The healthcare provider may perform a series of medical tests to rule out other bowel disorders, such as irritable bowel syndrome, Crohn's disease, or celiac disease, that may cause symptoms similar to those of ulcerative colitis.

How Is Ulcerative Colitis Treated?

A healthcare provider treats ulcerative colitis with:

- medications

- surgery

Which treatment a person needs depends on the severity of the disease and the symptoms. Each person experiences ulcerative colitis differently, so healthcare providers adjust treatments to improve the person's symptoms and induce, or bring about, remission.

Medications

While no medication cures ulcerative colitis, many can reduce symptoms. The goals of medication therapy are:

- inducing and maintaining remission

- improving the person's quality of life

Many people with ulcerative colitis require medication therapy indefinitely, unless they have their colon and rectum surgically removed.

Healthcare providers will prescribe the medications that best treat a person's symptoms:

- aminosalicylates

- corticosteroids

- immunomodulators

- biologics, also called anti-TNF therapies

- other medications

Depending on the location of the symptoms in the colon, healthcare providers may recommend a person take medications by:

- enema, which involves flushing liquid medication into the rectum using a special wash bottle. The medication directly treats inflammation of the large intestine.

- rectal foam—a foamy substance the person puts into the rectum like an enema. The medication directly treats inflammation of the large intestine.

- suppository—a solid medication the person inserts into the rectum to dissolve. The intestinal lining absorbs the medication.

- mouth.

- IV.

Aminosalicylates are medications that contain 5-aminosalicyclic acid (5-ASA), which helps control inflammation. Healthcare providers typically use aminosalicylates to treat people with mild or moderate symptoms or help people stay in remission. Aminosalicylates can be prescribed as an oral medication or a topical medication—by enema or suppository. Combination therapy—oral and rectal—is most effective, even in people with extensive ulcerative colitis. Aminosalicylates are generally well tolerated.

Aminosalicylates include:

- balsalazide

- mesalamine

- olsalazine

- sulfasalazine—a combination of sulfapyridine and 5-ASA

Some of the common side effects of aminosalicylates include:

- abdominal pain

- diarrhea

- headaches

- nausea

Healthcare providers may order routine blood tests for kidney function, as aminosalicylates can cause a rare allergic reaction in the kidneys.

Corticosteroids, also known as steroids, help reduce the activity of the immune system and decrease inflammation. Healthcare providers prescribe corticosteroids for people with more severe symptoms and people who do not respond to aminosalicylates. Healthcare providers do not typically prescribe corticosteroids for long-term use.

Corticosteroids are effective in bringing on remission; however, studies have not shown that the medications help maintain long-term remission. Corticosteroids include:

- budesonide

- hydrocortisone

- methylprednisone

- prednisone

Side effects of corticosteroids include:

- acne

- a higher chance of developing infections

- bone mass loss

- death of bone tissue

- high blood glucose

- high blood pressure

- mood swings

- weight gain

People who take budesonide may have fewer side effects than with other steroids.

Immunomodulators reduce immune system activity, resulting in less inflammation in the colon. These medications can take several weeks to 3 months to start working. Immunomodulators include:

- azathioprine

- 6-mercaptopurine, or 6-MP

Healthcare providers prescribe these medications for people who do not respond to 5-ASAs. People taking these medications may have the following side effects:

- abnormal liver tests

- feeling tired

- infection

- low white blood cell count, which can lead to a higher chance of infection

- nausea and vomiting

- pancreatitis

- slightly increased chance of lymphoma

- slightly increased chance of nonmelanoma skin cancers

Healthcare providers routinely test blood counts and liver function of people taking immunomodulators. People taking these medications should also have yearly skin cancer exams.

People should talk with their healthcare provider about the risks and benefits of immunomodulators.

Biologics—including adalimumab, golimumab, infliximab, and vedolizumab—are medications that target a protein made by the immune system called tumor necrosis factor (TNF). These medications decrease inflammation in the large intestine by neutralizing TNF. Anti-TNF therapies work quickly to bring on remission, especially in people who do not respond to other medications. Infliximab and vedolizumab are given through an IV; adalimumab and golimumab are given by injection.

Healthcare providers will screen patients for tuberculosis and hepatitis B before starting treatment with anti-TNF medications.

Side effects of anti-TNF medications may include:

- a higher chance of developing infections—especially tuberculosis or fungal infection

- skin cancer—melanoma

- psoriasis

Other medications to treat symptoms or complications may include:

- acetaminophen for mild pain. People with ulcerative colitis should avoid using ibuprofen, naproxen, and aspirin since these medications can make symptoms worse.

- antibiotics to prevent or treat infections.

- loperamide to help slow or stop diarrhea. In most cases, people only take this medication for short periods of time since it can increase the chance of developing megacolon. People should check with a healthcare provider before taking loperamide, because those with significantly active ulcerative colitis should not take this medication.

- cyclosporine—healthcare providers prescribe this medication only for people with severe ulcerative colitis because of the side effects. People should talk with their healthcare provider about the risks and benefits of cyclosporine.

Surgery

Some people will need surgery to treat their ulcerative colitis when they have:

- colon cancer

- dysplasia, or precancerous cells in the colon

- complications that are life threatening, such as megacolon or bleeding

- no improvement in symptoms or condition despite treatment

- continued dependency on steroids

- side effects from medications that threaten their health

Removal of the entire colon, including the rectum, "cures" ulcerative colitis. A surgeon performs the procedure at a hospital. A surgeon can perform two different types of surgery to remove a patient's colon and treat ulcerative colitis:

- proctocolectomy and ileostomy

- proctocolectomy and ileoanal reservoir

Full recovery from both operations may take 4 to 6 weeks.

Proctocolectomy and ileostomy. A proctocolectomy is surgery to remove a patient's entire colon and rectum. An ileostomy is a stoma, or opening in the abdomen, that a surgeon creates from a part of the ileum—the last section of the small intestine. The surgeon brings the end of the ileum through an opening in the patient's abdomen and attaches it to the skin, creating an

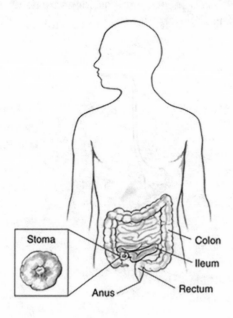

Figure 41.2. Ileostomy

opening outside of the patient's body. The stoma most often is located in the lower part of the patient's abdomen, just below the beltline.

A removable external collection pouch, called an ostomy pouch or ostomy appliance, connects to the stoma and collects intestinal contents outside the patient's body. Intestinal contents pass through the stoma instead of passing through the anus. The stoma has no muscle, so it cannot control the flow of intestinal contents, and the flow occurs whenever peristalsis occurs. Peristalsis is the movement of the organ walls that propels food and liquid through the GI tract.

People who have this type of surgery will have the ileostomy for the rest of their lives.

Proctocolectomy and ileoanal reservoir. An ileoanal reservoir is an internal pouch made from the patient's ileum. This surgery is a common alternative to an ileostomy and does not have a permanent stoma. Ileoanal reservoir is also known as a J-pouch, a pelvic pouch, or an ileoanal pouch anastamosis. The ileoanal reservoir connects the ileum to the anus. The surgeon preserves the outer muscles of the patient's rectum during the proctocolectomy. Next, the surgeon creates the ileal pouch and attaches it to the end of the rectum. Waste is stored in the pouch and passes through the anus.

After surgery, bowel movements may be more frequent and watery than before the procedure. People may have fecal incontinence—the accidental passing of solid or liquid stool or mucus from the rectum. Medications can be used to control pouch function. Women may be infertile following the surgery.

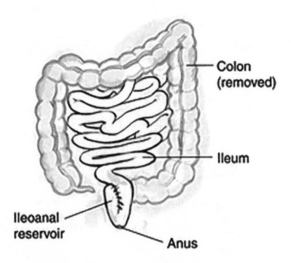

Figure 41.3. Ileoanal Reservoir

Many people develop pouchitis in the ileoanal reservoir. Pouchitis is an irritation or inflammation of the lining of the ileoanal reservoir. A healthcare provider treats pouchitis with antibiotics. Rarely, pouchitis can become chronic and require long-term antibiotics or other medications.

The surgeon will recommend one of the operations based on a person's symptoms, severity of disease, expectations, age, and lifestyle. Before making a decision, the person should get as much information as possible by talking with:

- healthcare providers

- enterostomal therapists, nurses who work with colon-surgery patients

- people who have had one of the surgeries

Patient-advocacy organizations can provide information about support groups and other resources.

What Are The Complications Of Ulcerative Colitis?

Complications of ulcerative colitis can include:

- rectal bleeding

- dehydration and malabsorbtion

- changes in bones

- inflammation in other areas of the body

- megacolon

Ulcerative Colitis And Colon Cancer

People with ulcerative colitis may be more likely to develop colon cancer when:

- ulcerative colitis affects the entire colon

- a person has ulcerative colitis for at least 8 years

- inflammation is ongoing

- people also have primary sclerosing cholangitis, a condition that affects the liver

- a person is male

People who receive ongoing treatment and remain in remission may reduce their chances of developing colon cancer. People with ulcerative colitis should talk with their healthcare provider about how often they should get screened for colon cancer. Screening can include colonoscopy with biopsies or a special dye spray called chromoendoscopy.

Healthcare providers may recommend colonoscopy every 1 to 3 years for people with ulcerative colitis who have:

- the disease in one-third or more or of their colon

- had ulcerative colitis for 8 years

Such screening does not reduce a person's chances of developing colon cancer. Instead, screening can help diagnose cancer early and improve chances for recovery. Surgery to remove the entire colon eliminates the risk of colon cancer.

Chapter 42

Eczema

Eczema is a term for several different types of skin swelling. Eczema is also called dermatitis. Most types cause dry, itchy skin and rashes on the face, inside the elbows and behind the knees, and on the hands and feet. Scratching the skin can cause it to turn red, and to swell and itch even more.

Eczema is not contagious. The cause is not known. It is likely caused by both genetic and environmental factors. Eczema may get better or worse over time, but it is often a long-lasting disease. People who have it may also develop hay fever and asthma.

The most common type of eczema is atopic dermatitis. It is most common in babies and children but adults can have it too. As children who have atopic dermatitis grow older, this problem may get better or go away. But sometimes the skin may stay dry and get irritated easily.

Treatments may include medicines, skin creams, light therapy, and good skin care. You can prevent some types of eczema by avoiding:

- Things that irritate your skin, such as certain soaps, fabrics, and lotions

- Stress

- Things you are allergic to, such as food, pollen, and animals

About This Chapter: Text in this chapter begins with excerpts from "Eczema," MedlinePlus, National Institutes of Health (NIH), August 15, 2016; Text beginning with the heading "Who Gets Atopic Dermatitis?" is excerpted from "Fast Facts About Atopic Dermatitis," National Institute of Arthritis and Musculoskeletal and Skin Diseases (NIAMS), November 2014. Reviewed October 2017.

Who Gets Atopic Dermatitis?

Atopic dermatitis is most common in babies and children. But it can happen to anyone. People who live in cities and dry climates may be more likely to get this disease. When children with atopic dermatitis grow older, this problem can improve or go away. But the skin may stay dry and easy to irritate. At other times, atopic dermatitis is a problem in adulthood.

You can't "catch" the disease or give it to other people.

Other Types Of Skin Problems

Atopic dermatitis is often called eczema. "Eczema" is a term for many kinds of skin problems. Atopic dermatitis is the most common kind of eczema. Other types include:

- **Allergic contact eczema.** The skin gets red, itchy, and weepy because it touches something that the immune system knows is foreign, like poison ivy.

- **Contact eczema.** The skin has redness, itching, and burning in one spot because it has touched something allergy-causing, like an acid, cleaner, or other chemical.

- **Dyshidrotic eczema.** The skin on the palms of hands and soles of the feet is irritated and has clear, deep blisters that itch and burn.

- **Neurodermatitis.** Scaly patches on the head, lower legs, wrists, or forearms are caused by a localized itch (such as an insect bite).

- **Nummular eczema.** The skin has coin-shaped spots of irritation. The spots can be crusted, scaling, and very itchy.

- **Seborrheic eczema.** This skin has yellowish, oily, scaly patches on the scalp, face, and sometimes other parts of the body.

- **Stasis dermatitis.** The skin is irritated on the lower legs, most often from a blood flow problem.

What Causes Atopic Dermatitis?

The cause of atopic dermatitis is not known. It is likely caused by both genetic (runs in the family) and environmental factors. People with atopic dermatitis may go on to develop hay fever and asthma.

How Is Atopic Dermatitis Diagnosed?

Diagnosis is based on the symptoms. Each person has his or her own mix of symptoms that can change over time. Doctors will ask for a medical history to:

- Learn about your symptoms
- Know when symptoms occur
- Rule out other diseases
- Look for causes of symptoms

Doctors also may ask about:

- Other family members with allergies
- Whether you have conditions such as hay fever or asthma
- Whether you have been around something that might bother the skin
- Sleep problems
- Foods that may lead to skin flares
- Treatments you have had for other skin problems
- Use of steroids or medicine

There isn't a certain test that can be used to check for this disease. But you may be tested for allergies by a dermatologist (skin doctor) or allergist (allergy doctor).

Things That Make Atopic Dermatitis Worse

Irritants and allergens can make atopic dermatitis worse.

Irritants are things that may cause the skin to be red and itchy or to burn. They include:

- Wool or manmade fibers
- Soaps and cleaners
- Some perfumes and makeup
- Substances such as chlorine, mineral oil, or solvents
- Dust or sand
- Cigarette smoke

Allergens are allergy-causing substances from foods, plants, animals, or the air. Common allergens are:

- Eggs, peanuts, milk, fish, soy products, and wheat

- Dust mites

- Mold

- Pollen

- Dog or cat dander

Stress, anger, and frustration can make atopic dermatitis worse, but they haven't been shown to cause it. Skin infections, temperature, and climate can also lead to skin flares. Other things that can lead to flares are:

- Not using enough lubricants after a bath

- Low humidity in winter

- Dry year-round climate

- Long or hot baths and showers

- Going from sweating to being chilled

- Bacterial infections

How Is Atopic Dermatitis Treated?

Treatment works best when the patient, family members, and the doctor work together. Treatment plans are based on:

- Age

- Symptoms

- General health

You need to carefully follow the treatment plan. Try to notice what is or isn't helpful. Symptoms usually improve with the right skin care and lifestyle changes.

Atopic dermatitis treatment goals are to heal the skin and prevent flares. Your doctor will help you:

- Develop a good skin care routine

- Avoid things that lead to flares

- Treat symptoms when they occur

You and your family members should watch for changes in the skin to find out what treatments help the most.

Medications for atopic dermatitis include:

- Skin creams or ointments that control swelling and lower allergic reactions

- Corticosteroids

- Antibiotics to treat infections caused by bacteria

- Antihistamines that make people sleepy to help stop nighttime scratching

- Drugs that suppress the immune system.

Other treatments include:

- Light therapy

- A mix of light therapy and a drug called psoralen

- Skin care that helps heal the skin and keep it healthy

- Protection from allergens

Atopic Dermatitis And Vaccination Against Smallpox

People with atopic dermatitis should not get the smallpox vaccine. It may cause serious problems in people with atopic dermatitis.

What Research Is Being Done On Atopic Dermatitis?

Research is being done into what causes atopic dermatitis, and how it can be managed, treated, and prevented.

Research includes:

- Genetics

- Biochemical changes in skin and white blood cells

- Immune factors
- Light therapy
- New medications
- Supplements, herbs, and plant extracts

Chapter 43

Hair Loss

What Is Alopecia Areata?

Alopecia areata is a disease that affects the hair follicles, which are part of the skin from which hairs grow. In most cases, hair falls out in small, round patches about the size of a quarter. Many people with the disease get only a few bare patches. Some people may lose more hair. Rarely, the disease causes total loss of hair on the head or complete loss of hair on the head, face, and body.

Who Gets Alopecia Areata?

Anyone can have alopecia areata. It often begins in childhood. There is a slightly increased risk of having the disease if you have a close family member with the disease.

What Causes Alopecia Areata?

Alopecia areata is an autoimmune disease. Normally the immune system protects the body against infection and disease. In an autoimmune disease, the body's immune system mistakenly attacks some part of your own body. In alopecia areata, the immune system attacks the hair follicles.

The cause is not known. Scientists think that a person's genes may play a role. For people whose genes put them at risk for the disease, some type of trigger starts the attack on the hair follicles. The triggers may be a virus or something in the person's environment.

About This Chapter: This chapter includes text excerpted from "Fast Facts About Alopecia Areata," National Institute of Arthritis and Musculoskeletal and Skin Diseases (NIAMS), April 2015.

Will My Hair Ever Grow Back?

There is every chance that your hair will grow back, but it may fall out again. No one can tell you when it might fall out or grow back. You may lose more hair, or your hair loss may stop. The hair you have lost may or may not grow back. Even a person who has lost all of his hair may grow all of his hair back. The disease varies from person to person.

How Is Alopecia Areata Treated?

There is no cure for alopecia areata. There are no drugs approved to treat it. Doctors may use medicines approved for other diseases to help hair grow back. However, none of these treatments prevent new patches of hair loss or cure the disease. Talk to your doctor about the treatment that is best for you.

How Will Alopecia Areata Affect My Life?

Alopecia areata does not make you feel pain and does not make you feel sick. You can't give it to others. People who have the disease are, for the most part, healthy in other ways. Alopecia areata will not shorten your life, and it should not affect activities such as going to school, working, marrying, raising a family, playing sports, and exercising.

How Can I Cope With The Effects Of This Disease

Living with hair loss can be hard. There are many things you can do to cope with the effects of this disease, including:

- Learning as much as you can about the disease.

- Talking with others who are dealing with the disease.

- Learning to value yourself for who you are, not for how much hair you have or don't have.

- Talking with a counselor, if necessary, to help build a positive self-image.

Here are some things you can use to reduce the physical dangers or discomforts of lost hair:

- Use sunscreens for the scalp, face, and all exposed skin.

- Wear eyeglasses (or sunglasses) to protect eyes from sun, and from dust and debris, when eyebrows or eyelashes are missing.

- Wear wigs, caps, or scarves to protect the scalp from the sun and keep the head warm.

- Apply antibiotic ointment inside the nostrils to help keep germs out of the nose when nostril hair is missing.

Here are some things you can do to reduce the disease's effects on your looks:

- Try wearing a wig, hairpiece, scarf, or cap.

- Use a hair-colored powder, cream, or crayon applied to the scalp for small patches of hair loss to make the hair loss less obvious.

- Use an eyebrow pencil to mask missing eyebrows.

What Research Is Being Done On Alopecia Areata?

Researchers are seeking a better understanding of the disease. Scientists are studying:

- Genes

- Hair follicle development

- Immune treatments

- Stem cells in the skin

- Medications

Part Five
Stress Management

Chapter 44

Importance Of Managing Stress

The Basics

Not all stress is bad. But chronic (ongoing) stress can lead to health problems.

Preventing and managing chronic stress can lower your risk for serious conditions like heart disease, obesity, high blood pressure, and depression.

You can prevent or reduce stress by:

- Planning ahead
- Deciding which tasks need to be done first
- Preparing for stressful events

Some stress is hard to avoid. You can find ways to manage stress by:

- Noticing when you feel stressed
- Taking time to relax
- Getting active and eating healthy
- Talking to friends and family

What Are The Signs Of Stress?

When people are under stress, they may feel:

- Worried
- Angry

About This Chapter: This chapter includes text excerpted from "Manage Stress," Office of Disease Prevention and Health Promotion (ODPHP), U.S. Department of Health and Human Services (HHS), June 26, 2017.

- Irritable
- Depressed
- Unable to focus

Stress also affects the body. Physical signs of stress include:

- Headaches
- Back pain
- Problems sleeping
- Upset stomach
- Weight gain or loss
- Tense muscles
- Frequent or more serious colds

What Causes Stress?

Change is often a cause of stress. Even positive changes, like having a baby or getting a job promotion, can be stressful. Stress can be short-term or long-term.

What Are The Benefits Of Managing Stress?

Over time, chronic stress can lead to health problems. Managing stress can help you:

- Sleep well
- Control your weight
- Get sick less often
- Feel better faster when you do get sick
- Have less neck and back pain
- Be in a better mood
- Get along better with family and friends

Take Action!

Being prepared and feeling in control of your situation might help lower your stress. Follow these 9 tips for preventing and managing stress.

1. **Plan your time.**

   Think ahead about how you are going to use your time. Write a to-do list and figure out what's most important—then do that thing first. Be realistic about how long each task will take.

2. **Prepare yourself.**

    Prepare ahead of time for stressful events like a job interview or a hard conversation with a loved one.

    - Stay positive.

    - Picture what the room will look like and what you will say.

    - Have a back-up plan.

3. **Relax with deep breathing or meditation.**

    Deep breathing and meditation are 2 ways to relax your muscles and clear your mind.

    - Find out how easy it is to use deep breathing to relax

    - Try meditating for a few minutes today

4. **Relax your muscles.**

    Stress causes tension in your muscles. Try stretching or taking a hot shower to help you relax.

5. **Get active.**

    Regular physical activity can help prevent and manage stress. It can also help relax your muscles and improve your mood.

    - Aim for 2 hours and 30 minutes a week of physical activity. Try going for a bike ride or taking a walk.

    - Be sure to exercise for at least 10 minutes at a time.

    - Do strengthening activities—like crunches or lifting weights—at least 2 days a week.

6. **Eat healthy.**

    Give your body plenty of energy by eating healthy foods—including vegetables, fruits, and lean sources of protein.

7. **Drink alcohol only in moderation.**

    Avoid using alcohol or other drugs to manage stress. If you choose to drink, drink only in moderation. This means no more than 1 drink a day for women and no more than 2 drinks a day for men.

8. **Talk to friends and family.**

Tell your friends and family if you are feeling stressed. They may be able to help.

9. **Get help if you need it.**

Stress is a normal part of life. But if your stress doesn't go away or keeps getting worse, you may need help. Over time, stress can lead to serious problems like depression, anxiety, or PTSD (posttraumatic stress disorder).

- If you are feeling down or hopeless, talk to a doctor about depression.

- If you are feeling anxious, find out how to get help for anxiety.

- If you have lived through an unsafe event, find out about treatment for PTSD.

A mental health professional (like a psychologist or social worker) can help treat these conditions with talk therapy (called psychotherapy) or medicine.

Lots of people need help dealing with stress—it's nothing to be ashamed of!

Chapter 45

Coping With Stress

Coping With Stress

Everyone—adults, teens, and even children—experiences stress at times. Stress can be beneficial by helping people develop the skills they need to cope with and adapt to new and potentially threatening situations throughout life. However, the beneficial aspects of stress diminish when it is severe enough to overwhelm a person's ability to take care of themselves and family. Using healthy ways to cope and getting the right care and support can put problems in perspective and help stressful feelings and symptoms subside.

Sometimes after experiencing a traumatic event that is especially frightening—including personal or environmental disasters, or being threatened with an assault—people have a strong and lingering stress reaction to the event. Strong emotions, jitters, sadness, or depression may all be part of this normal and temporary reaction to the stress of an overwhelming event.

Common reactions to a stressful event can include:

- Disbelief, shock, and numbness

- Feeling sad, frustrated, and helpless

- Fear and anxiety about the future

- Feeling guilty

- Anger, tension, and irritability

- Difficulty concentrating and making decisions

About This Chapter: This chapter includes text excerpted from "Violence Prevention," Centers for Disease Control and Prevention (CDC), October 2, 2015.

- Crying

- Reduced interest in usual activities

- Wanting to be alone

- Loss of appetite

- Sleeping too much or too little

- Nightmares or bad memories

- Reoccurring thoughts of the event

- Headaches, back pains, and stomach problems

- Increased heart rate, difficulty breathing

- Smoking or use of alcohol or drugs

Tips To Deal With Stress

Prepare yourself for stressful situations. If something is coming up that's making you nervous, doing a little homework in advance can make a big difference. Nervous about talking to your teacher or coach? Practice what you're going to say in front of a mirror. Got a big game or performance coming up? Picture yourself nailing it.

When you're really upset, try using the stop-breathe-think method. Take a timeout—stop, take a deep breath, and think about what's going on. A short break from a stressful or upsetting situation can help you think more clearly and make a healthy decision about what to do next.

Reward yourself with fun. If you're feeling really stressed or sad, it can be tough to build fun activities into your life. Find ways to reward yourself—even small things like picking up your favorite magazine or listening to music can improve your mood. Choose an activity that you stopped doing when you started dipping, or try something new that you've always wanted to do.

Healthy Ways To Cope With Stress

Feeling emotional and nervous or having trouble sleeping and eating can all be normal reactions to stress. Engaging in healthy activities and getting the right care and support can put problems in perspective and help stressful feelings subside in a few days or weeks. Some tips for beginning to feel better are:

- Take care of yourself.

- Eat healthy, well-balanced meals

- Exercise on a regular basis

- Get plenty of sleep

- Give yourself a break if you feel stressed out

- Talk to others. Share your problems and how you are feeling and coping with a parent, friend, counselor, doctor, or pastor.

- Avoid drugs and alcohol. Drugs and alcohol may seem to help with the stress. In the long run, they create additional problems and increase the stress you are already feeling.

- Take a break. If your stress is caused by a national or local event, take breaks from listening to the news stories, which can increase your stress.

Recognize when you need more help If problems continue or you are thinking about suicide, talk to a psychologist, social worker, or professional counselor.

Helping Youth Cope With Stress

Because of their level of development, children and adolescents often struggle with how to cope well with stress. Youth can be particularly overwhelmed when their stress is connected to a traumatic event—like a natural disaster (earthquakes, tornados, or wildfires), family loss, school shootings, or community violence. Parents and educators can take steps to provide stability and support that help young people feel better.

Tips For Parents

It is natural for children to worry, especially when scary or stressful events happen in their lives. Talking with children about these stressful events and monitoring what children watch or hear about the events can help put frightening information into a more balanced context. Some suggestions to help children cope are:

- **Maintain a normal routine.** Helping children wake up, go to sleep, and eat meals at regular times provide them a sense of stability. Going to school and participating in typical after-school activities also provide stability and extra support.

- **Talk, listen, and encourage expression.** Create opportunities to have your children talk, but do not force them. Listen to your child's thoughts and feelings and share some of yours. After a traumatic event, it is important for children to feel like they can share their feelings and to know that their fears and worries are understandable. Keep these conversations going by asking them how they feel in a week, then in a month, and so on.

- **Watch and listen.** Be alert for any change in behavior. Are children sleeping more or less? Are they withdrawing from friends or family? Are they behaving in any way out of the ordinary? Any changes in behavior, even small changes, may be signs that the child is having trouble coming to terms with the event and may support.

- **Reassure.** Stressful events can challenge a child's sense of physical and emotional safety and security. Take opportunities to reassure your child about his or her safety and well-being and discuss ways that you, the school, and the community are taking steps to keep them safe.

- **Connect with others.** Make an on-going effort to talk to other parents and your child's teachers about concerns and ways to help your child cope. You do not have to deal with problems alone-it is often helpful for parents, schools, and health professionals to work together to support and ensuring the wellbeing of all children in stressful times.

Tips For Kids And Teen

After a traumatic or violent event, it is normal to feel anxious about your safety and security. Even if you were not directly involved, you may worry about whether this type of event may someday affect you. How can you deal with these fears? Start by looking at the tips below for some ideas.

- **Talk to and stay connected to others.** This connection might be your parent, another relative, a friend, neighbor, teacher, coach, school nurse, counselor, family doctor, or member of your church or temple. Talking with someone can help you make sense out of your experience and figure out ways to feel better. If you are not sure where to turn, call your local crisis intervention center or a national hotline.

- **Get active.** Go for a walk, play sports, write a play or poem, play a musical instrument, or join an after-school program. Volunteer with a community group that promotes nonviolence or another school or community activity that you care about. Trying any of these can be a positive way to handle your feelings and to see that things are going to get better.

- **Take care of yourself.** As much as possible, try to get enough sleep, eat right, exercise, and keep a normal routine. It may be hard to do, but by keeping yourself healthy you will be better able to handle a tough time.

- **Take information breaks.** Pictures and stories about a disaster can increase worry and other stressful feelings. Taking breaks from the news, Internet, and conversations about the disaster can help calm you down.

Chapter 46

Talk To Your Parents Or Other Adults

Strong emotions like fear, sadness, or other symptoms of depression are normal, as long as they are temporary and don't interfere with daily activities. If these emotions last too long or cause other problems, it's a different story.

Sometimes stress can be good. It can help you develop skills needed to manage potentially threatening situations. Stress can be harmful, however, when it is prolonged or severe enough to make you feel overwhelmed and out of control.

Talking To Your Parents About Emotional Problems

It takes courage to tell a parent or guardian that you are having trouble with your feelings. But adults can help you through tough times, and it's important to get the support you need.

When you're ready, try to find a time when you won't get interrupted. You may even need to schedule a time to talk. Try saying something like, "Mom and Dad, I have something I'd like to talk about. Can we sit and talk after dinner?"

If talking seems too hard, it might be easier to write your thoughts. A letter, an email, or even a text message can get the conversation going. Try something as simple as "I've been feeling anxious" or "I'm worried I might be depressed." Or you might just say, "I need your help."

About This Chapter: Text in this chapter begins with excerpts from "Coping With Stress," Centers for Disease Control and Prevention (CDC), December 7, 2016; Text under the heading "Talking To Your Parents About Emotional Problems" is excerpted from "Talking To Your Parents About Emotional Problems," girlshealth.gov, Office on Women's Health (OWH), January 7, 2015.

Tips For Self-Care

The best ways to manage stress in hard times are through self-care.

- **Avoid drugs and alcohol.** They may seem to be a temporary fix to feel better, but in the long run drugs and alcohol can create more problems and add to your stress—instead of taking it away.
- **Find support.** Seek help from a partner, family member, friend, counselor, doctor, or clergyperson. Having someone with a sympathetic, listening ear and sharing about your problems and stress really can lighten the burden.
- **Connect socially.** After a stressful event, it is easy isolate yourself. Make sure that you are spending time with loved ones. Consider planning fun activities with your partner, children, or friends.
- **Take care of yourself.**
- Eat a healthy, well-balanced diet
- Exercise regularly
- Get plenty of sleep
- Give yourself a break if you feel stressed out—for example, treat yourself to a therapeutic massage
- Maintain a normal routine
- **Stay active.** You can take your mind off your problems with activities like helping a neighbor, volunteering in the community, and taking the dog on a long walk. These can be positive ways to cope with stressful feelings.

Keep in mind that if your parents or you get upset, you can continue the conversation over time. If they ask a question about your feelings that you can't answer, you might say you'll think about it and will talk more later.

If you think you definitely can't talk to your parents or guardians, reach out to another trusted adult. This might be a school counselor, teacher, religious leader, school nurse, or doctor. Definitely don't give up. You deserve to feel better!

Chapter 47

Going To A Therapist

Lots of teens have some kind of emotional problem. In fact, almost half of U.S. teens will have a mental health problem before they turn 18. The good news is that therapy can really help.

Sometimes, people are embarrassed or afraid to see a therapist. But getting help from a therapist because you're feeling sad or anxious is really not different from seeing a doctor because you broke a bone. In fact, you can feel proud for being brave enough to do what you need to do to get your life back on track.

What Is Therapy?

Therapy is when you talk about your problems with someone who is a professional counselor, such as a psychiatrist, psychologist, or social worker. Therapy sometimes is called psychotherapy. That is because it helps with your psychology—the mental and emotional parts of your life.

If you are going through a rough time, talking to a caring therapist can be a great relief. A therapist can help you cope with sadness, worry, and other strong or scary feelings. Here are some other ways therapy can help:

- It can teach you specific skills for handling difficult situations, such as problems with your family or school.

- It can help you find healthy ways to deal with stress or anger.

- It can teach you how to build healthy relationships.

About This Chapter: This chapter includes text excerpted from "Going To Therapy," girlshealth.gov, Office on Women's Health (OWH), January 7, 2015.

- It can help you figure out how to think about things in more positive ways.

- It can help you figure out how to boost your self-confidence.

- It can help you decide where you want to go in life and how to deal with any obstacles that may come up along the way.

Therapy may feel great right away, or it might feel strange at first. It can take a little time getting used to talking with someone new about your problems. But therapists are trained to listen well, and they want to help.

As time goes on, you should feel comfortable with your therapist. If you don't feel comfortable, or if you think you're not getting better, tell your parent or guardian. Another therapist or type of therapy might work better.

Therapists protect people's privacy. They can share what you say only in very special cases, such as if they think you are in danger. If you're concerned, though, ask about the privacy policy. It's important to feel like you can tell the truth in therapy. It works best if you are honest about any problems you're facing, including problems with drugs or alcohol or any behaviors that can hurt your body or mind.

Just because you start to see a therapist doesn't mean that you will see one forever. You should be able to learn skills that let you handle your problems on your own. Sometimes, a few sessions are all you need to learn skills and feel better.

Want to know more about therapy? You can get more info on seeing a therapist External link, including whether or not to tell your friends.

Why Do Teens Go For Therapy?

Many young people develop mental health conditions, like depression, eating disorders, or anxiety disorders. If you have a mental health problem, remember there are treatments that work, and you can feel better. Also, some teens go to therapy to get help through a tough time, like their parents' getting divorced or having too much stress at school.

If you feel out of control, or you feel like a mental health problem keeps you from enjoying life, get help. Reach out to a parent or guardian or another trusted adult.

What Should I Do To Get Started With Therapy?

If you need help finding a therapist, you can start by talking to your doctor, school nurse, or school counselor. If your family has insurance, the insurance company can tell you which therapists are covered under your plan.

If you need help paying for therapy, you can ask a parent or guardian if they have health insurance that might help pay for therapy.

What Are Some Kinds Of Therapy?

There are different kinds of therapy to help you feel better. The best treatment depends on the type of problem that you are facing.

You may have one-on-one talk therapy. This is when you talk to a therapist alone. Or you may join group therapy, where you work with a therapist and other people who are having similar issues. You may also do art therapy, where you paint or draw.

One kind of talk therapy that tends to work well for depression, anxiety, and several other problems is cognitive behavioral therapy. This type of therapy teaches you how to think and act in healthier ways.

Sometimes, your therapist will suggest that you take medicine in addition to therapy, which often can be a helpful combination.

What About Online Support Groups?

There are lots of support groups available on the Internet, including ones to help you handle your feelings. Chat rooms and other online options may help you feel less alone. But if you are having trouble coping, it's important to work with a therapist or other mental health professional.

Remember to be careful about getting info online. Some people use the Internet to promote unhealthy behaviors, like cutting and dangerous eating habits.

Chapter 48

Handle Your Anger

Anger can be so overwhelming. You may feel like you could smash something or someone. Everyone feels angry at times. That's natural. What matters is how you handle your anger.

Because anger is so intense, it can be pretty scary and confusing. Plus, you may have learned that being angry isn't "nice."

What Are Reasons To Control Anger?

It's important to figure out how to handle anger for a lot of reasons.

If you don't find healthy ways to express your anger, your physical health can suffer. Strong anger or anger that lasts a long time can be stressful. Stress can lead to health problems such as heart disease, high blood pressure, backaches, and stomach trouble.

If you don't handle your anger well, you run the risk of developing emotional problems, like depression or eating disorders. You also may get in trouble in school and have a hard time building strong, healthy relationships. And you may not feel as good about yourself as you'd like.

How Can I Deal With Anger?

Everyone is different, so everyone will find different ways to handle anger.

About This Chapter: This chapter includes text excerpted from "Feeling Angry," girlshealth.gov, Office on Women's Health (OWH), January 7, 2015.

Here are some suggestions to get you started:

- **Think about why you want to change.**

  You'll have your own thoughts on this, but you can check out some common reasons to control anger above. You might even write down your reasons and look at them at times to keep you motivated.

- **Identify problems and solutions.**

  See if you can figure out what exactly is bothering you. Then see if you can find ways to solve the problem. If a person is bothering you, maybe you can avoid that person. Or maybe the two of you can agree to negotiate and compromise.

- **Notice how your body feels when you are angry.**

  Feelings in your body may be the first signs that you're angry. Your stomach might hurt, for example, or your breathing might change. The sooner you know that you're starting to steam, the sooner you can work to calm down. You might take nice, deep breaths or count to 10 slowly.

- **Try to see the other person's side if you are angry at him or her.**

  Is your little sister being a pest by constantly hanging around? Maybe it's because she thinks you're great. Can you remember feeling that way about someone? Seeing things through her eyes can help you be more patient.

- **Express yourself calmly.**

  If you have a healthy relationship with someone, you should be able to tell them how you feel. Just wait until you cool off enough to have a respectful conversation.

- **Take responsibility for your actions.**

  If you feel like other people do things that "make" you angry, keep in mind that only you are in charge of you. Plan ahead when you know you will be seeing someone who bothers you. Try to think of some ideas that will help keep you calm.

What If I Have A Lot Of Anger Inside?

It's great to have a plan for how to handle anger when it comes up. You can also work on ways to keep anger under control on a regular basis.

Here are some suggestions:

- **Talk to someone you trust.** It can be a relief just to share how you're feeling. You can talk with a friend, a relative, a teacher, or anyone you trust. You also can work with a therapist to understand your feelings better and find ways to handle anger.

- **Get moving.** Physical activity can burn off extra energy and help you feel more relaxed.

- **Write in a journal.** Writing can be a great way to let your feelings out. It also may give you a chance to explore what is really going on. Often, other emotions, such as hurt or fear, are underneath the anger. Knowing what's really going on can help calm the anger.

- **Let music soothe you.** Listen to your favorite tunes, sing in the shower, play an instrument, or write a song about how you feel.

- **Get creative.** Drawing, painting, or creating something can be a great release.

- **Get good sleep.** It's easier to stay calm and think straight when you're well-rested.

The Anger Control Plan

- Take a time out (formal or informal).
- Talk to a friend (someone you trust).
- Use the Conflict Resolution Model to express anger.
- Exercise (take a walk, go to the gym, etc.).
- Attend 12-step meetings.
- Explore primary feelings beneath the anger.

(Source: "Managing Anger," Substance Abuse and Mental Health Services Administration (SAMHSA).)

What If My Anger Starts To Get Out Of Control?

If you feel like your anger is boiling over, make sure to keep yourself and others around you safe. Here are some things you can do:

- **Get out.** Remove yourself from a tense situation. But don't drive—driving when angry can be dangerous. Take a walk, which is a great way to burn off extra energy.

- **Choose safe ways to calm down.** You might take deep breaths, repeat a calming word, or imagine a calm place. Don't drink or use drugs to handle anger.

- **Get help.** If you feel you are a danger to yourself or others, call 911 or go to the closest hospital emergency department. It's important to get help right away.

Chapter 49

Body Image And Self-Esteem

Do you wish you could lose weight, get taller, or develop faster? It's pretty common to worry a little about how your body looks, especially when it's changing. You can learn about body image and ways to take control of yours.

What Is Body Image?

Body image is how you think and feel about your body. It includes whether you think you look good to other people.

Body image is affected by a lot of things, including messages you get from your friends, family, and the world around you. Images we see in the media definitely affect our body image even though a lot of media images are changed or aren't realistic.

Why does body image matter? Your body image can affect how you feel about yourself overall. For example, if you are unhappy with your looks, your self-esteem may start to go down. Sometimes, having body image issues or low self-esteem may lead to depression, eating disorders, or obesity.

How Can I Deal With Body Image Issues?

Everyone has something they would like to change about their bodies. But you'll be happier if you focus on the things you like about your body—and your whole self. Need some help? Check out some tips:

About This Chapter: Text in this chapter begins with excerpts from "Having Body Image Issues," girlshealth.gov, Office on Women's Health (OWH), January 7, 2015; Text beginning with the heading "What Is Self-Esteem?" is excerpted from "Self-Esteem And Self-Confidence," girlshealth.gov, Office on Women's Health (OWH), January 7, 2015.

- **List your great traits.** If you start to criticize your body, tell yourself to stop. Instead, think about what you like about yourself, both inside and out.

- **Know your power.** Hey, your body is not just a place to hang your clothes! It can do some truly amazing things. Focus on how strong and healthy your body can be.

- **Treat your body well.** Eat right, sleep tight, and get moving. You'll look and feel your best—and you'll be pretty proud of yourself too.

- **Give your body a treat.** Take a nice bubble bath, do some stretching, or just curl up on a comfy couch. Do something soothing.

- **Mind your media.** Try not to let models and actresses affect how you think you should look. They get lots of help from makeup artists, personal trainers, and photo fixers. And advertisers often use a focus on thinness to get people to buy stuff. Don't let them mess with your mind!

- **Let yourself shine.** A lot of how we look comes from how we carry ourselves. Feeling proud, walking tall, and smiling big can boost your beauty—and your mood.

- **Find fab friends.** Your best bet is to hang out with people who accept you for you! And work with your friends to support each other.

If you can't seem to accept how you look, talk to an adult you trust. You can get help feeling better about your body.

Stressing About Body Changes

During puberty and your teen years, your body changes a lot. All those changes can be hard to handle. They might make you worry about what other people think of how you look and about whether your body is normal. If you have these kinds of concerns, you are not alone.

Here are some common thoughts about changing bodies.

- Why am I taller than most of the boys my age?

- Why haven't I grown?

- Am I too skinny?

- Am I too fat?

- Will others like me now that I am changing?

- Are my breasts too small?

- Are my breasts too large?
- Why do I have acne?
- Do my clothes look right on my body?
- Are my hips getting bigger?

If you are stressed about your body, you may feel better if you understand why you are changing so fast—or not changing as fast as your friends.

During puberty, you get taller and see other changes in your body, such as wider hips and thighs. Your body will also start to have more fat compared to muscle than before. Each young woman changes at her own pace, and all of these changes are normal.

What Are Serious Body Image Problems?

If how your body looks bothers you a lot and you can't stop thinking about it, you could have body dysmorphic disorder, or BDD.

People with BDD think they look ugly even if they have a small flaw or none at all. They may spend many hours a day looking at flaws and trying to hide them. They also may ask friends to reassure them about their looks or want to have a lot of cosmetic surgery. If you or a friend may have BDD, talk to an adult you trust, such as a parent or guardian, school counselor, teacher, doctor, or nurse. BDD is an illness, and you can get help.

What Is Self-Esteem?

Self-esteem has to do with the **value** and **respect** you have for yourself. Simply put, it's your opinion of yourself.

If you have healthy self-esteem, you feel good about yourself and are proud of what you can do. Having healthy self-esteem can help you feel positive overall. And it can make you brave enough to tackle some serious challenges, like trying out for a school play or standing up to a bully.

If you have low self-esteem, you may not think very highly of yourself. Of course, it's normal to feel down about yourself sometimes. But if you feel bad about yourself more often than good, you may have low self-esteem.

How can low self-esteem hurt? Low self-esteem may stop you from doing things you want to do or from speaking up for yourself. Low self-esteem may even lead you to try to feel better in unhealthy ways, like using drugs or alcohol. Also, some people may start to feel so sad or hopeless about themselves that they develop mental health problems like depression and eating disorders.

A lot of things can affect self-esteem. These include how others treat you, your background and culture, and experiences at school. For example, being put down by your boyfriend, classmates, or family or being bullied can affect how you see yourself. But one of the biggest influences on your self-esteem is… you!

What Is Self-Confidence?

Self-confidence is a little different from self-esteem. Self-confidence has to do with what you think about your skills and abilities.

Self-confidence often comes from trying new things, like speaking more in class or trying out for an afterschool activity. Does that sound a little stressful? That's normal! As you try new things, you will gain confidence in spite of your fears. In fact, that's what real self-confidence is—your belief that you will be fine even in the face of obstacles.

Rate Your Self-Esteem And Self-Confidence

If you have healthy self-esteem and self-confidence, you probably will agree with some or most of the following statements:

- I feel good about who I am.

- I am proud of what I can do, but don't need to show off.

- I know there are some things that I'm good at and some things I need to improve.

- I feel it is okay if I win or if I lose.

- I usually think, "I can do this," before I do something.

- I am eager to learn new things.

- I can handle criticism.

- I like to try to do things without help, but I don't mind asking for help if I need it.

- I like myself.

If some of the items on this checklist are true for you, congrats! You're on the right track.

If you have low self-esteem and self-confidence, you probably will agree with some or most of the following statements:

- I can't do anything well.

- I have no friends.

- I do not like to try new things.

- I get really upset about making mistakes.

- I'm not as nice, pretty, or smart as the other girls in my class.

- I don't like it when people say nice things about me.

- I get very upset when people criticize me.

- I feel better if I put other people down.

- I don't know what I'm good at.

- I usually think, "I can't do this," before I do something.

- I don't like myself.

If many of the items on this list apply to you, try some ways to raise your self-esteem. It's no fun to be hard on yourself, and you can work to stop. Remember, everyone brings something unique to the world.

Boost Your Self-Esteem And Self-Confidence

Do you want to feel better about yourself? You can learn how to build self-esteem and raise your self-confidence. Try these tips:

- Check out new activities. You'll feel proud for stretching your wings. Does trying something new on your own seem too scary? Maybe see if a friend will go along.

- Be your own BFF. Make a list of things you love about you. Are you friendly, funny, creative, or hard-working, for example?

- Celebrate your successes. Try to really enjoy your achievements. Record them in a journal, tell your friends, or hang up pictures or other reminders.

- Tell your inner critic to be quiet. If you have a mean thought about yourself, see if you can change it to something positive instead. For example, if you think, "I'm dumb," try remembering a time you did something smart.

- Don't compare yourself to others. Someone else may have tons of online friends or a "great" body. But everyone has strengths and weaknesses.

- Practice being assertive. Try to express your thoughts, opinions, and needs. It feels great to know you can speak up for yourself! (Of course, you want to do this without stomping on other people's feelings.)

- Find ways to feel like you're contributing. It feels great to help. You might do chores at home or volunteer in your community.

- Set realistic goals. Aim for a goal that you think you can reach. Then make a plan for how to get there. If you pick something very hard, you may get frustrated and quit.

- Forgive yourself when you fail. Nobody is perfect. The important thing is to learn from your mistakes. And it's good to know you can pick yourself up and keep going!

- Find true friends. Hang out with people who make you feel good about yourself. Real friends like you for you.

- Honor your background. It can be great to feel proud of who you are and where you come from. Read about exploring your culture and what girls have to say about their unique identities.

- If you try working on your self-esteem for a while and still don't feel good about yourself, reach out for help. Talk to a parent or guardian, doctor, school counselor, school nurse, teacher, or other trusted adult. An adult may be able to suggest other things you can try, and it may help just to talk about how you're feeling. Also, sometimes low self-esteem can increase your risk for depression and other emotional problems. An adult you trust could help you get treatment if you need it.

(Source: "Boost Your Self-Esteem And Self-Confidence," Office on Women's Health (OWH).)

Chapter 50

Exercise Is Wise

You may wonder if being physically active is really worth the time and effort. Well, lots of girls think so! They know being active is a great way to have fun and hang out with friends.

What Being Active Does For Your Mental Health?

Did you know being physically active can affect how good you feel? It also can affect how well you do your tasks, and even how pleasant you are to be around. That's partly because physical activity gets your brain to make "feel-good" chemicals called endorphins. Regular physical activity may help you by:

- Reducing stress

- Improving sleep

- Boosting your energy

- Reducing symptoms of anxiety and depression

- Increasing your self-esteem

- Making you feel proud for taking good care of yourself

- Improving how well you do at school

What Being Active Does For Your Body?

Being physically active is great for your muscles, heart, and lungs.

About This Chapter: This chapter includes text excerpted from "Why Physical Activity Is Important," girlshealth. gov, Office on Women's Health (OWH), March 27, 2015.

It may even help with nasty PMS symptoms! Some other possible benefits of activity include:

- **Building strong bones.** Your body creates the most bone when you are a kid and a teen. Learn more about how to build great bones.

- **Promoting a healthy weight.** Obesity is a serious problem among kids in the United States. It can lead to problems with your sleep, knees, heart, emotions, and more, but exercise can help.

- **Helping avoid diabetes.** A lot more young people are getting diabetes than ever before. Regular physical activity can help prevent one type of diabetes.

- **Building healthy habits.** If you get used to being active now, you will more likely keep it up when you're older. You'll thank yourself later!

- **Fighting cancer.** Research shows that exercise may help protect against certain kinds of cancer, including breast cancer.

- **Helping prevent high blood pressure.** The number of kids with high blood pressure is growing. High blood pressure makes your heart and arteries work extra hard to pump blood. It also puts you at risk for things like kidney and eye disease.

Are you worried that exercise will bulk you up? Exercising won't give you big, bulging muscles. It takes a very intense weightlifting program to get a bodybuilder look. And exercise and other forms of physical activity can help if you need to lose weight or want to stay a healthy weight.

Fitness Basics

Being active may not be as hard as you think. You definitely don't need a gym membership or fancy equipment. Here are some key points to help you build a strong, healthy body:

- **You should aim for at least 60 minutes of activity every day.** You can be active for an hour all at once. Or, you can do a few shorter activities, such as walking to school and playing ball later. (And at least 60 minutes is the right amount from the time you're 6 years old until you turn 18.)

- **You need a mix of different kinds of activities.** Learn about the main types of activity, how they help, and great ways to do them.

- **Most of your 60 minutes should be spent on aerobic activity.** Aerobic activity is anything that gets your heart pumping, such as dancing, running, or swimming laps.

- **How hard you exercise matters, too.** You can learn how to measure your workout to see if it is light, medium, or intense.

- **Focus on fun.** Pick activities you enjoy so you'll be more likely to keep doing them. Also, avoid boredom through variety. We've got ideas for ways to shake up your routine.

- **Start slowly if you haven't been active in a while.** Start with what you can do. Over time, add more days to your activity routine or more time each day. You'll get there!

- **If you have a disability, you should still aim for 60 minutes of activity each day.** Talk with your doctor about what exercises are right for you.

Chapter 51

Yoga

Yoga in its full form combines physical postures, breathing exercises, meditation, and a distinct philosophy. There are numerous styles of yoga. Hatha yoga, commonly practiced in the United States and Europe, emphasizes postures, breathing exercises, and meditation. Hatha yoga styles include Ananda, Anusara, Ashtanga, Bikram, Iyengar, Kripalu, Kundalini, Vini-yoga, and others.

Side Effects And Risks

- Yoga is generally low-impact and safe for healthy people when practiced appropriately under the guidance of a well-trained instructor.

- Overall, those who practice yoga have a low rate of side effects, and the risk of serious injury from yoga is quite low. However, certain types of stroke as well as pain from nerve damage are among the rare possible side effects of practicing yoga.

- Women who are pregnant and people with certain medical conditions, such as high blood pressure, glaucoma (a condition in which fluid pressure within the eye slowly increases and may damage the eye's optic nerve), and sciatica (pain, weakness, numbing, or tingling that may extend from the lower back to the calf, foot, or even the toes), should modify or avoid some yoga poses.

About This Chapter: Text in this chapter begins with excerpts from "Yoga: In Depth," National Center for Complementary and Integrative Health (NCCIH), September 19, 2017; Text under the heading "Practicing Yoga" is excerpted from "BAM! Body And Mind—Yoga Activity Card," Centers for Disease Control and Prevention (CDC), May 9, 2015.

Practicing Yoga

Did you know that yoga has been around for more than 5,000 years? Today, you see lots of super stars and athletes practicing yoga, but it's a great activity for anyone! No matter what other activities you participate in, yoga can strengthen your abilities by increasing flexibility, staying power (endurance), and your ability to focus.

Lots of physical activities build your muscles and strength, but many times other parts of your body are left out. Because yoga is a full body workout, it can help to check any imbalance in your muscles.

In addition, yoga strengthens, tones, and stretches your muscles, helping to increase your flexibility. If your body is flexible you will be less likely to get injured.

Most yoga practices focus on physical postures called "asanas," breathing exercises called "pranayama," and meditation to bring your body and mind together through slow, careful movements. But, there's more to it than that! Yoga leads to improved physical fitness, increased ability to concentrate, and decreased stress. Yoga is an activity that helps both your body and mind work a little better.

When To Practice

Yoga can fit easily into your schedule—taking 10–15 minutes each day to practice can make a difference (just make sure to wait at least two to three hours after you've eaten!). Yoga is a perfect way to chill out and take some time just for yourself! So, set aside a special time each day and relax, release, and rejuvenate!

Where To Practice

Find a quiet spot where you won't be distracted. Look for a level area that is large enough for you to stretch upwards as well as to the sides for standing and floor positions or stretches.

How To Practice

Always warm up! Plan a well-rounded workout that includes lots of different positions from all of the major muscle groups (arms, legs, abs, back, and chest). Most importantly, remember to breathe! It's a good idea to start with several arm stretches over your head and deep breaths. Inhale when you try upward and expanded movements, and exhale during downward or forward bending motions.

Concentrate on each position—move slowly making controlled movements until you feel your muscles tensing and resisting (you should feel your muscles stretching, not straining). Each pose in yoga is an experiment, so go slowly and listen to your body. Know when you are pushing yourself too hard or need to challenge yourself a little more.

Last but not least, remember to take 5–10 minutes to relax your body at the end of your workout. This will help to prevent sore muscles and is a way to unwind your body.

Practice Yoga Safely

Follow these tips to minimize your risk of injury:

- Talk to your care provider
- Find a trained and experienced yoga practitioner
- Adapt poses to your individual needs and abilities

(Source: "Yoga As A Complementary Health Approach," National Center for Complementary and Integrative Health (NCCIH).)

Chapter 52

Tai Chi

What Are Tai Chi And Qi Gong?

Tai chi and qi gong are centuries-old, related mind and body practices. They involve certain postures and gentle movements with mental focus, breathing, and relaxation. The movements can be adapted or practiced while walking, standing, or sitting. In contrast to qi gong, tai chi movements, if practiced quickly, can be a form of combat or self-defense.

What The Science Says About The Effectiveness Of Tai Chi And Qi Gong?

Research findings suggest that practicing tai chi may improve balance and stability in older people and those with Parkinson's, reduce pain from knee osteoarthritis, help people cope with fibromyalgia and back pain, and promote quality of life and mood in people with heart failure and cancer. There's been less research on the effects of qi gong, but some studies suggest it may reduce chronic neck pain (although results are mixed) and pain from fibromyalgia. Qi gong also may help to improve general quality of life.

Both also may offer psychological benefits, such as reducing anxiety. However, differences in how the research on anxiety was conducted make it difficult to draw firm conclusions about this.

About This Chapter: Text beginning with the heading "What Are Tai Chi And Qi Gong?" is excerpted from "Tai Chi And Qi Gong: In Depth," National Center for Complementary and Integrative Health (NCCIH), October 2016; Text under the heading "Five Tips: What You Should Know About Tai Chi For Health" is excerpted from "5 Tips: What You Should Know About Tai Chi For Health," National Center for Complementary and Integrative Health (NCCIH), September 24, 2015.

Falling And Balance

Exercise programs, including tai chi, may reduce falling and the fear of falling in older people. Tai chi also may be more effective than other forms of exercise for improving balance and stability in people with Parkinson disease.

- A 2012 review determined that tai chi, as well as other group- and home-based activity programs (which often include balance and strength-training exercises) effectively reduced falling in older people, and tai chi significantly reduced the risk of falling. But the reviewers also found that tai chi was less effective in older people who were at higher risk of falling.

- Fear of falling can have a serious impact on an older person's health and life. In a 2014 review, researchers suggested that various types of exercise, including tai chi, may reduce the fear of falling among older people.

- Findings from a 2012 clinical trial with 195 people showed that practicing tai chi improved balance and stability better than resistance training or stretching in people with mild-to-moderate Parkinson's disease. A 2014 follow-up analysis showed that people who practiced tai chi were more likely to continue exercising during the 3 months following the study compared with those who participated in resistance training or stretching.

For Pain (Knee Osteoarthritis, Fibromyalgia, Chronic Neck Pain, And Back Pain)

There's some evidence that practicing tai chi may help people manage pain associated with knee osteoarthritis (a breakdown of cartilage in the knee that allows leg bones to rub together), fibromyalgia (a disorder that causes muscle pain and fatigue), and back pain. Qi gong may offer some benefit for chronic neck pain, but results are mixed.

Knee Osteoarthritis

- Results of a small National Center for Complementary and Integrative Health (NCCIH)-funded clinical trial involving 40 participants with knee osteoarthritis suggested that practicing tai chi reduced pain and improved function better than an education and stretching program.

- An analysis of seven small and moderately-sized clinical studies concluded that a 12-week course of tai chi reduced pain and improved function in people with this condition.

Fibromyalgia

- Results from a small 2010 NCCIH-supported clinical trial suggested that practicing tai chi was more effective than wellness education and stretching in helping people with fibromyalgia sleep better and cope with pain, fatigue, and depression. After 12 weeks, those who practiced tai chi also had better scores on a survey designed to measure a person's ability to carry out certain daily activities such as walking, housecleaning, shopping, and preparing a meal. The benefits of tai chi also appeared to last longer.

- A small 2012 NCCIH-supported trial suggested that combining tai chi movements with mindfulness allowed people with fibromyalgia to work through the discomfort they may feel during exercise, allowing them to take advantage of the benefits of physical activity.

- Results of a 2012 randomized clinical trial with 100 participants suggested that practicing qi gong reduced pain and improved sleep, the ability to do daily activities, and mental function. The researchers also observed that most improvements were still apparent after 6 months.

Chronic Neck Pain

Research results on the effectiveness of qi gong for chronic neck pain are mixed, but the people who were studied and the way the studies were done were quite different.

- A 2009 clinical study by German researchers showed no benefit of qi gong or exercise compared with no therapy in 117 elderly adults (mostly women) with, on average, a 20-year history of chronic neck pain. Study participants had 24 exercise or qi gong sessions over 3 months.

- In a 2011 study, some of the same researchers observed that qi gong was just as effective as exercise therapy (and both were more effective than no therapy) in relieving neck pain in the 123 middle-aged adults (mostly women) who had chronic neck pain for an average of 3 years. Exercise therapy included throwing and catching a ball, rowing and climbing movements, arm swinging, and stretching, among other activities. People in the study had 18 exercise or qi gong sessions over 6 months.

Back Pain

In people who had low-back pain for at least 3 months, a program of tai chi exercises reduced their pain and improved their functioning.

For Mental Health And Cognitive Function

While a range of research has suggested that exercise helps reduce depression and anxiety, the role of tai chi and qi gong for these and other mental health problems is less clear. However, there is evidence that tai chi may boost brain function and reasoning ability in older people.

- NCCIH-supported research suggested that practicing tai chi may help reduce stress, anxiety, and depression, and also improve mood and self-esteem. However, in their 2010 review, which included 40 studies with more than 3,800 participants, the researchers noted that they couldn't develop firm conclusions because of differences in study designs.

- In a 2010 NCCIH-supported review, researchers found that the results from 29 studies with more than 2,500 participants didn't offer clear evidence about the effectiveness of tai chi and qi gong on such psychological factors as anxiety, depression, stress, mood, and self-esteem. But the researchers noted that most of these studies weren't looking primarily at psychological distress and didn't intentionally recruit participants with mental health issues.

- Results from another NCCIH-supported review published in 2014 suggested that practicing tai chi may enhance the ability to reason, plan, remember, and solve problems in older people without evidence of significant cognitive impairment. The data also indicated that tai chi boosted cognitive ability in people who showed signs of mild cognitive impairment to dementia, but to a lesser degree than in those with no signs of cognitive impairment.

For Quality Of Life

Much research suggests that physical activity enhances quality of life. Health providers who treat people with cancer often recommend exercise to reduce illness-related fatigue and improve quality of life. Some studies also suggest that physical activity helps people with heart disease and other chronic illnesses.

Cancer

Research results indicated that practicing qi gong may improve quality of life, mood, fatigue, and inflammation in adults with different types of cancer, compared with those receiving usual care. However, the researchers suggested that the attention received by the qi gong participants may have contributed to the positive study findings.

Heart Disease

- Regular practice of tai chi may improve quality of life and mood in people with chronic heart failure, according to a 2011 clinical trial funded by NCCIH.

- Results from a small study suggested that practicing tai chi improved the ability to exercise and may be an option as cardiac rehabilitation for people who have had a heart attack.

Other

A NCCIH-supported research review examined the effects of tai chi and qi gong on the quality of life of adults who were healthy, elderly, were breast cancer or stroke survivors, or had a chronic disease. The analysis suggested that practicing tai chi or qi gong may improve quality of life in healthy and chronically ill people.

Five Tips: What You Should Know About Tai Chi For Health

Here are five things to know about tai chi for health.

1. Research findings suggest that practicing tai chi may improve balance and stability in older people and reduce the risk of falls. There is also some evidence that tai chi may improve balance impairments in people with mid-to-moderate Parkinson disease.

2. There is some evidence to suggest that practicing tai chi may help people manage chronic pain associated with knee osteoarthritis and help people with fibromyalgia sleep better and cope with pain, fatigue, and depression.

3. Although tai chi has not been shown to have an effect on the disease activity of rheumatoid arthritis (e.g., tender and swollen joints, activities of daily living), there is some evidence that tai chi may improve lower extremity (ankle) range of motion in people with rheumatoid arthritis. It is not known if tai chi improves pain associated with rheumatoid arthritis or quality of life.

4. Tai chi may promote quality of life and mood in people with heart failure and cancer. Tai chi also may offer psychological benefits, such as reducing anxiety. However, differences in how the research on anxiety was conducted make it difficult to draw firm conclusions about this.

5. Take charge of your health—talk with your healthcare providers about any complementary health approaches you use. Together, you can make shared, well-informed decisions.

Chapter 53

Use Your Senses To Relieve Stress

There are countless techniques for preventing stress. Yoga and meditation work wonders for improving our coping skills. But who can take a moment to chant or meditate during a job interview or a disagreement with your spouse? For these situations, you need something more immediate and accessible. That's when quick stress relief comes to the rescue.

The speediest way to stamp out stress is by engaging one or more of your senses—your sense of sight, sound, taste, smell, touch, or movement—to rapidly calm and energize yourself.

Remember exploring your senses in elementary school? Grownups can take a tip from grade school lessons by revisiting the senses and learning how they can help us prevent stress overload. Use the following exercises to identify the types of stress-busting sensory experiences that work quickly and effectively for you.

Sights

If you're a visual person, try to manage and relieve stress by surrounding yourself with soothing and uplifting images. You can also try closing your eyes and imagining the soothing images. Here are a few visually-based activities that may work as quick stress relievers:

- Look at a cherished photo or a favorite memento.

- Bring the outside indoors; buy a plant or some flowers to enliven your space.

- Enjoy the beauty of nature–a garden, the beach, a park, or your own backyard.

- Surround yourself with colors that lift your spirits.

About This Chapter: This chapter includes text excerpted from "The Basics Of Quick Stress Relief: Engage Your Senses," U.S. Department of Veterans Affairs (VA), May 12, 2015.

- Close your eyes and picture a situation or place that feels peaceful and rejuvenating.

Sound

Are you sensitive to sounds and noises? Are you a music lover? If so, stress-relieving exercises that focus on your auditory sense may work particularly well. Experiment with the following sounds, noting how quickly your stress levels drop as you listen.

- Sing or hum a favorite tune. Listen to uplifting music.

- Tune in to the soundtrack of nature-crashing waves, the wind rustling the trees, birds singing.

- Buy a small fountain, so you can enjoy the soothing sound of running water in your home or office.

- Hang wind chimes near an open window.

Smell And Scents

If you tend to zone out or freeze when stressed, surround yourself with smells that are energizing and invigorating. If you tend to become overly agitated under stress, look for scents that are comforting and calming.

- Light a scented candle or burn some incense.

- Lie down in sheets scented with lavender.

- Smell the roses-or another type of flower.

- Enjoy the clean, fresh air in the great outdoors.

- Spritz on your favorite perfume or cologne.

Touch

Experiment with your sense of touch, playing with different tactile sensations. Focus on things you can feel that are relaxing and renewing. Use the following suggestions as a jumping off point:

- Wrap yourself in a warm blanket.

- Pet a dog or cat.

- Hold a comforting object (a stuffed animal, a favorite memento).

- Soak in a hot bath.

- Give yourself a hand or neck massage.
- Wear clothing that feels soft against your skin.

Taste

Slowly savoring a favorite treat can be very relaxing, but mindless stress eating will only add to your stress and your waistline. The key is to indulge your sense of taste mindfully and in moderation. Eat slowly, focusing on the feel of the food in your mouth and the taste on your tongue:

- Chew a piece of sugarless gum.
- Indulge in a small piece of dark chocolate.
- Sip a steaming cup of coffee or tea or a refreshing cold drink.
- Eat a perfectly ripe piece of fruit.
- Enjoy a healthy, crunchy snack (celery, carrots, or trail mix).

Movement

If you tend to shut down when you're under stress, stress-relieving activities that get you moving may be particularly helpful. Anything that engages the muscles or gets you up and active can work. Here are a few suggestions:

- Run in place or jump up and down.
- Dance around.
- Stretch or roll your head in circles.
- Go for a short walk.
- Squeeze a rubbery stress ball.

The Power Of Imagination

Sensory rich memories can also quickly reduce stress. After drawing upon your sensory toolbox becomes habit, another approach is to learn to simply imagine vivid sensations when stress strikes. Believe it or not, the mere memory of your baby's face will have the same calming or energizing effects on your brain as seeing her photo. So if you can recall a strong sensation, you'll never be without access to your quick stress relief toolbox.

Chapter 54

Meditation

What Is Meditation?

Meditation is a mind and body practice that has a long history of use for increasing calmness and physical relaxation, improving psychological balance, coping with illness, and enhancing overall health and wellbeing. Mind and body practices focus on the interactions among the brain, mind, body, and behavior.

There are many types of meditation, but most have four elements in common: a quiet location with as few distractions as possible; a specific, comfortable posture (sitting, lying down, walking, or in other positions); a focus of attention (a specially chosen word or set of words, an object, or the sensations of the breath); and an open attitude (letting distractions come and go naturally without judging them).

What The Science Says About The Effectiveness Of Meditation

Many studies have investigated meditation for different conditions, and there's evidence that it may reduce blood pressure as well as symptoms of irritable bowel syndrome and flare-ups in people who have had ulcerative colitis. It may ease symptoms of anxiety and depression, and may help people with insomnia.

About This Chapter: This chapter includes text excerpted from "Meditation: In Depth," National Center for Complementary and Integrative Health (NCCIH), April 2016.

For Anxiety, Depression, And Insomnia

- A 2014 literature review of 47 trials in 3,515 participants suggests that mindfulness meditation programs show moderate evidence of improving anxiety and depression. But the researchers found no evidence that meditation changed health-related behaviors affected by stress, such as substance abuse and sleep.

- A review of 36 trials found that 25 of them reported better outcomes for symptoms of anxiety in the meditation groups compared to control groups.

- In a small, NCCIH-funded study, 54 adults with chronic insomnia learned mindfulness-based stress reduction (MBSR), a form of MBSR specially adapted to deal with insomnia (mindfulness-based therapy for insomnia, or MBTI), or a self-monitoring program. Both meditation-based programs aided sleep, with MBTI providing a significantly greater reduction in insomnia severity compared with MBSR.

---

8 Things To Know About Meditation For Health

For people who suffer from cancer symptoms and treatment side effects, mind-body therapies, such as meditation, have been shown to help relieve anxiety, stress, fatigue, and general mood and sleep disturbances, thus improving their quality of life.

There is some evidence that meditation may reduce blood pressure.

- A growing body of evidence suggests that meditation-based programs may be helpful in reducing common menopausal symptoms.
- There is moderate evidence that meditation improves symptoms of anxiety.
- Some studies suggest that mindfulness meditation helps people with irritable bowel syndrome (IBS), but there's not enough evidence to draw firm conclusions.
- Overall, there is not enough evidence to know whether mind-body practices are as effective as other treatments to help people quit smoking.
- There isn't enough evidence to support the use of meditation for attention deficit hyperactivity disorder (ADHD).
- Meditation is generally considered to be safe for healthy people.

(Source: "8 Things To Know About Meditation For Health," National Center for Complementary and Integrative Health (NICCH).)

Meditation And The Brain

Some research suggests that meditation may physically change the brain and body and could potentially help to improve many health problems and promote healthy behaviors.

- In a study, researchers compared brain images from 50 adults who meditate and 50 adults who don't meditate. Results suggested that people who practiced meditation for many years have more folds in the outer layer of the brain. This process (called gyrification) may increase the brain's ability to process information.

- A 2013 review of three studies suggests that meditation may slow, stall, or even reverse changes that take place in the brain due to normal aging.

- Results from a NCCIH-funded study suggest that meditation can affect activity in the amygdala (a part of the brain involved in processing emotions), and that different types of meditation can affect the amygdala differently even when the person is not meditating.

- Research about meditation's ability to reduce pain has produced mixed results. However, in some studies scientists suggest that meditation activates certain areas of the brain in response to pain.

What The Science Says About Safety And Side Effects Of Meditation

- Meditation is generally considered to be safe for healthy people.

- People with physical limitations may not be able to participate in certain meditative practices involving movement. People with physical health conditions should speak with their healthcare providers before starting a meditative practice, and make their meditation instructor aware of their condition.

- There have been rare reports that meditation could cause or worsen symptoms in people with certain psychiatric problems like anxiety and depression. People with existing mental health conditions should speak with their healthcare providers before starting a meditative practice, and make their meditation instructor aware of their condition.

Chapter 55

Relaxation Techniques

What Are Relaxation Techniques?

Relaxation techniques include a number of practices such as progressive relaxation, guided imagery, biofeedback, self-hypnosis, and deep breathing exercises. The goal is similar in all: to produce the body's natural relaxation response, characterized by slower breathing, lower blood pressure, and a feeling of increased well-being.

Meditation and practices that include meditation with movement, such as yoga and tai chi, can also promote relaxation. You can find information about these practices elsewhere on the National Center for Complementary and Integrative Health (NCCIH) website.

Stress management programs commonly include relaxation techniques. Relaxation techniques have also been studied to see whether they might be of value in managing various health problems.

The Importance Of Practice

Relaxation techniques include the following:

Autogenic Training

In autogenic training, you learn to concentrate on the physical sensations of warmth, heaviness, and relaxation in different parts of your body.

About This Chapter: This chapter includes text excerpted from "Relaxation Techniques For Health," National Center for Complementary and Integrative Health (NCCIH), May 2016.

Biofeedback-Assisted Relaxation

Biofeedback techniques measure body functions and give you information about them so that you can learn to control them. Biofeedback-assisted relaxation uses electronic devices to teach you to produce changes in your body that are associated with relaxation, such as reduced muscle tension.

Deep Breathing Or Breathing Exercises

This technique involves focusing on taking slow, deep, even breaths.

Guided Imagery

For this technique, people are taught to focus on pleasant images to replace negative or stressful feelings. Guided imagery may be self-directed or led by a practitioner or a recording.

Progressive Relaxation

This technique, also called Jacobson relaxation or progressive muscle relaxation, involves tightening and relaxing various muscle groups. Progressive relaxation is often combined with guided imagery and breathing exercises.

Self-Hypnosis

In self-hypnosis programs, people are taught to produce the relaxation response when prompted by a phrase or nonverbal cue (called a "suggestion").

What The Science Says About The Effectiveness Of Relaxation Techniques

Researchers have evaluated relaxation techniques to see whether they could play a role in managing a variety of health conditions, including the following:

Anxiety

Studies have shown relaxation techniques may reduce anxiety in people with ongoing health problems such as heart disease or inflammatory bowel disease, and in those who are having medical procedures such as breast biopsies or dental treatment. Relaxation techniques have also been shown to be useful for older adults with anxiety.

On the other hand, relaxation techniques may not be the best way to help people with generalized anxiety disorder. Generalized anxiety disorder is a mental health condition, lasting for months or longer, in which a person is often worried or anxious about many things and finds it hard to control the anxiety. Studies indicate that long-term results are better in people with generalized anxiety disorder who receive a type of psychotherapy called cognitive-behavioral therapy than in those who are taught relaxation techniques.

Depression

An evaluation of 15 studies concluded that relaxation techniques are better than no treatment in reducing symptoms of depression but are not as beneficial as psychological therapies such as cognitive-behavioral therapy.

Fibromyalgia

- Studies of guided imagery for fibromyalgia have had inconsistent results.

- A 2013 evaluation of the research concluded that electromyographic (EMG) biofeedback, in which people are taught to control and reduce muscle tension, helped to reduce fibromyalgia pain, at least for short periods of time. However, EMG biofeedback didn't affect sleep problems, depression, fatigue, or health-related quality of life in people with fibromyalgia, and its long-term effects haven't been established.

Headache

- Biofeedback. Biofeedback has been studied for both tension headaches and migraines.

- An evaluation of high-quality studies concluded that there's conflicting evidence about whether biofeedback can relieve tension headaches.

- Studies have shown decreases in the frequency of migraines in people who were using biofeedback. However, it's unclear whether biofeedback is better than a placebo.

- Other Relaxation Techniques. Relaxation techniques other than biofeedback have been studied for tension headaches. An evaluation of high-quality studies found conflicting evidence on whether relaxation techniques are better than no treatment or a placebo. Some studies suggest that other relaxation techniques are less effective than biofeedback.

Heart Disease

In people with heart disease, studies have shown relaxation techniques can reduce stress and anxiety and may also have beneficial effects on physical measures such as heart rate.

High Blood Pressure

Stress can lead to a short-term increase in blood pressure, and the relaxation response has been shown to reduce blood pressure on a short-term basis, allowing people to reduce their need for blood pressure medication. However, it's uncertain whether relaxation techniques can have long-term effects on high blood pressure.

Insomnia

There's evidence that relaxation techniques can be helpful in managing chronic insomnia. Relaxation techniques can be combined with other strategies for getting a good night's sleep, such as maintaining a consistent sleep schedule; avoiding caffeine, alcohol, heavy meals, and strenuous exercise too close to bedtime; and sleeping in a quiet, cool, dark room.

Irritable Bowel Syndrome (IBS)

An evaluation of research results by the American College of Gastroenterology concluded that relaxation techniques have not been shown to help irritable bowel syndrome. However, other psychological therapies, including cognitive-behavioral therapy and hypnotherapy, are associated with overall symptom improvement in people with irritable bowel syndrome.

Menopause Symptoms

Relaxation techniques have been studied for hot flashes and other symptoms associated with menopause, but the quality of the research isn't high enough to allow definite conclusions to be reached.

Menstrual Cramps

Some research suggests that relaxation techniques may be beneficial for menstrual cramps, but definite conclusions can't be reached because of the small number of participants in the studies and the poor quality of some of the research.

Nausea

An evaluation of the research evidence concluded that some relaxation techniques, including guided imagery and progressive muscle relaxation, are likely to be effective in relieving nausea caused by cancer chemotherapy when used in combination with antinausea drugs.

Nightmares

Some studies have indicated that relaxation exercises may be an effective approach for nightmares of unknown cause and those associated with posttraumatic stress disorder. However, an assessment of many studies concluded that relaxation is less helpful than more extensive forms of treatment (psychotherapy or medication).

Pain

Evaluations of the research evidence have found promising but not conclusive evidence that guided imagery may help relieve some musculoskeletal pain (pain involving the bones or muscles) and other types of pain.

An analysis of data on hospitalized cancer patients showed that those who received integrative medicine therapies, such as guided imagery and relaxation response training, during their hospitalization had reductions in both pain and anxiety.

Pain In Children And Adolescents

A 2014 evaluation of the scientific evidence found that psychological therapies, which may include relaxation techniques as well as other approaches such as cognitive-behavioral therapy, can reduce pain in children and adolescents with chronic headaches or other types of chronic pain. The evidence is particularly promising for headaches: the effect on pain may last for several months after treatment, and the therapies also help to reduce anxiety.

Ringing In The Ears (Tinnitus)

Only a few studies have evaluated relaxation techniques for ringing in the ears. The limited evidence from these studies suggests that relaxation techniques might be useful, especially in reducing the intrusiveness of the problem.

Smoking Cessation

Limited evidence suggests that guided imagery may be a valuable tool for people who are working to quit smoking. In a study that compared the two techniques, autogenic training was found to be less effective than cognitive-behavioral therapy as a quit-smoking aid. However, this study involved patients in an alcohol detoxification program, so its results may not be applicable to other people.

Preliminary research suggests that a guided relaxation routine might help reduce cigarette cravings.

Temporomandibular Joint Dysfunction

Problems with the temporomandibular joint (the joint that connects the jaw to the side of the head) can cause pain and difficulty moving the jaw. A few studies have shown that programs that include relaxation techniques may help relieve symptoms of temporomandibular joint dysfunction.

What The Science Says About The Safety And Side Effects Of Relaxation Techniques

- Relaxation techniques are generally considered safe for healthy people. However, occasionally, people report negative experiences such as increased anxiety, intrusive thoughts, or fear of losing control.

- There have been rare reports that certain relaxation techniques might cause or worsen symptoms in people with epilepsy or certain psychiatric conditions, or with a history of abuse or trauma. People with heart disease should talk to their healthcare provider before doing progressive muscle relaxation.

Try Progressive Muscle Relaxation

Progressive Muscle Relaxation shows you how to relax your muscles through tension and release. This can help lower your overall tension and stress levels, and help you relax when you are feeling anxious. Practicing this exercise will help you learn what relaxation feels like, and to notice when you get tense during the day.

1. Plan to take about 15 minutes to do the exercise.

2. Find a quiet place where no one will disturb you.

3. First, apply muscle tension to a specific part of the body. Take a slow, deep breath and squeeze the muscles as hard as you can for about 5 seconds.

4. After about 5 seconds, quickly relax the tensed muscles. Exhale as you let all the tightness flow out of the tensed muscles. The muscles should feel loose as you relax them. It's very important for you to notice and focus on the difference between the tension and relaxation.

5. Stay relaxed for about 15 seconds, and then do the same thing for the next muscle group. Once you've gone through all of the muscle groups, take a moment to enjoy the relaxation.

(Source: "Practice Mindfulness And Relaxation," U.S. Department of Health and Human Services (HHS).)

NCCIH-Funded Research

NCCIH is supporting a variety of studies on relaxation techniques. Examples of topics currently being studied include:

- The use of relaxation techniques and other complementary approaches for back pain in real-world healthcare settings

- Guided imagery and relaxation response training for pain management in hospitalized patients

Who Teaches Relaxation Techniques?

A variety of professionals, including physicians, psychologists, social workers, nurses, and complementary health practitioners, may teach relaxation techniques. Also, people sometimes learn the simpler relaxation techniques on their own.

More To Consider

- If you have severe or long-lasting symptoms of any kind, see your healthcare provider. You might have a condition that needs to be treated promptly. For example, if depression or anxiety persists, it's important to seek help from a qualified healthcare professional.

- Tell all your healthcare providers about any complementary or integrative health approaches you use. Give them a full picture of what you do to manage your health. This will help ensure coordinated and safe care.

Chapter 56

Massage Therapy

What Is Massage Therapy?

The term "massage therapy" includes many techniques, and the type of massage given usually depends on your needs and physical condition.

- Massage therapy dates back thousands of years. References to massage appear in ancient writings from China, Japan, India, and Egypt.

- In general, massage therapists work on muscle and other soft tissue to help you feel better.

- In Swedish massage, the therapist uses long strokes, kneading, deep circular movements, vibration, and tapping.

- Sports massage combines techniques of Swedish massage and deep tissue massage to release chronic muscle tension. It's adapted to the needs of athletes.

- Myofascial trigger point therapy focuses on trigger points—areas that are painful when pressed and are associated with pain elsewhere in the body.

- Massage therapy is sometimes done using essential oils as a form of aromatherapy.

What The Science Says About The Effectiveness Of Massage

A lot of the scientific research on massage therapy is preliminary or conflicting, but much of the evidence points toward beneficial effects on pain and other symptoms associated with a

About This Chapter: This chapter includes text excerpted from "Massage Therapy For Health Purposes," National Center for Complementary and Integrative Health (NCCIH), June 2016.

number of different conditions. Much of the evidence suggests that these effects are short term and that people need to keep getting massages for the benefits to continue.

Researchers have studied the effects of massage for many conditions. Some that they have studied more extensively are the following

Pain

- A research review and National Center for Complementary and Integrative Health (NCCIH)-funded clinical trial concluded that massage may be useful for chronic low-back pain.

- Massage may help with chronic neck pain, a NCCIH-funded clinical trial reported.

- Massage may help with pain due to osteoarthritis of the knee, according to a 2012 NCCIH-funded study.

- Studies suggest that for women in labor, massage provided some pain relief and increased their satisfaction with other forms of pain relief, but the evidence isn't strong, a 2012 review concluded.

Cancer

Numerous research reviews and clinical studies have suggested that at least for the short term, massage therapy for cancer patients may reduce pain, promote relaxation, and boost mood.

However, the National Cancer Institute (NCI) urges massage therapists to take specific precautions with cancer patients and avoid massaging:

- Open wounds, bruises, or areas with skin breakdown

- Directly over the tumor site

- Areas with a blood clot in a vein

- Sensitive areas following radiation therapy.

Mental Health

- A meta-analysis of 17 clinical trials concluded that massage therapy may help to reduce depression.

- Brief, twice-weekly yoga and massage sessions for 12 weeks were associated with a decrease in depression, anxiety, and back and leg pain in pregnant women with depression, a NCCIH-funded clinical trial showed. Also, the women's babies weighed more than babies born to women who didn't receive the therapy.

- However, a research review concluded that there's not enough evidence to determine if massage helps pregnant mothers with depression.

- A review concluded that massage may help older people relax.

- For generalized anxiety disorder, massage therapy was no better at reducing symptoms than providing a relaxing environment and deep breathing lessons, according to a small, NCCIH-supported clinical trial.

Fibromyalgia

A review concluded that massage therapy may help temporarily reduce pain, fatigue, and other symptoms associated with fibromyalgia, but the evidence is not definitive. The authors noted that it's important that the massage therapist not cause pain.

Headaches

Clinical trials on the effects of massage for headaches are preliminary and only somewhat promising.

HIV/AIDS

Massage therapy may help improve the quality of life for people with HIV or AIDS, a review of four small clinical trials concluded.

Infant Care

Massaging preterm infants using moderate pressure may improve weight gain, a 2010 review suggested. We don't have enough evidence to know if massage benefits healthy infants who are developing normally, a 2013 review determined.

Other Conditions

Researchers have studied massage for the following but it's still unclear if it helps:
- Behavior of children with autism or autism spectrum disorders
- Immune function in women with breast cancer
- Anxiety and pain in patients following heart surgery

- Quality of life and glucose levels in people with diabetes

- Lung function in children with asthma.

What The Science Says About The Safety And Side Effects Of Massage Therapy

Massage therapy appears to have few risks when performed by a trained practitioner. However, massage therapists should take some precautions in people with certain health conditions.

- In some cases, pregnant women should avoid massage therapy. Talk with your healthcare provider before getting a massage if you're pregnant.

- People with some conditions such as bleeding disorders or low blood platelet counts should avoid having forceful and deep tissue massage. People who take anticoagulants (also known as blood thinners) also should avoid them. Massage should not be done in any potentially weak area of the skin, such as wounds.

- Deep or intense pressure should not be used over an area where the patient has a tumor or cancer, unless approved by the patient's healthcare provider.

NCCIH-Funded Research

NCCIH-sponsored studies have investigated the effects of massage on a variety of conditions including:

- The effects of an 8-week course of Swedish massage compared to usual care on pain and function in adults with osteoarthritis of the knee

- Whether massage helps with generalized anxiety disorder

- The effect of massage therapy on cancer-related fatigue

- How massage therapy and progressive muscle relaxation compare for reducing chronic low-back pain in patients referred from primary care practices

- The frequency and length of massages needed to address neck pain.

Training, Licensing, And Certification

In the United States, 44 states and the District of Columbia regulate massage therapists. Cities, counties, or other local governments also may regulate massage. Training standards and requirements for massage therapists vary greatly by state and locality.

Most states that regulate massage therapists require them to have a minimum of 500 hours of training from an accredited training program. The National Certification Board for Therapeutic Massage and Bodywork certifies practitioners who pass a national examination and fulfill other requirements.

More To Consider

- Do not use massage therapy to replace conventional care or to postpone seeing a healthcare provider about a medical problem.

- If you have a medical condition and are unsure whether massage therapy would be appropriate for you, discuss your concerns with your healthcare provider, who may also be able to help you select a massage therapist.

- Ask about the training, experience, and credentials of the massage therapist you are considering. Also ask about the number of treatments that might be needed, the cost, and insurance coverage.

- For more tips on finding a complementary health practitioner, such as a massage therapist, see the National Center for Complementary and Integrative Health's (NCCIH) Web page How To Find a Complementary Health Practitioner.

- Tell all your healthcare providers about any complementary and integrative health approaches you use. Give them a full picture of what you do to manage your health. This will ensure coordinated and safe care.

Chapter 57

Spirituality

What Is Spirituality?

Spirituality is a personal experience with many definitions. Spirituality might be defined as "an inner belief system providing an individual with meaning and purpose in life, a sense of the sacredness of life, and a vision for the betterment of the world." Other definitions emphasize "a connection to that which transcends the self." The connection might be to God, a higher power, a universal energy, the sacred, or to nature. Researchers in the field of spirituality have suggested three useful dimensions for thinking about one's spirituality:

- Beliefs
- Spiritual practices
- Spiritual experiences

Currently in the United States, opinion surveys consistently find that most people endorse a belief in God or higher power. In a Gallup Poll 86 percent of respondents indicated a belief in God, while only 6 percent stated they did not believe in God. Many of these individuals would describe religion or spirituality as the most important source of strength and direction for their lives. Because spirituality plays such a significant and central role in the lives of many people, it is likely to be affected by trauma, and in turn to affect the survivor's reaction to the trauma.

Historically, there have been differences between the beliefs of scientists and health-care practitioners and those of the general population. For example, one study indicated

About This Chapter: This chapter includes text excerpted from "Spirituality And Trauma: Professionals Working Together," U.S. Department of Veterans Affairs (VA), May 26, 2016.

that only 66 percent of psychologists report a "belief in God." These differences in viewpoint may contribute to the lack of research on spirituality. The beliefs and training experiences of practitioners may also influence whether and how spirituality is incorporated into therapy.

Relationship Of Trauma To Spirituality

Evidence suggests that trauma can produce both positive and negative effects on the spiritual experiences and perceptions of individuals. For example, depression and loneliness can lead to feelings of abandonment and loss of faith in God. These effects may change as time passes and a person moves further away from the acute phase of trauma recovery.

On the positive side, some individuals experience increased appreciation of life, greater perceived closeness to God, increased sense of purpose in life, and enhanced spiritual well-being even following devastating events such as disasters and rape. For others, trauma can be associated with loss of faith, diminished participation in religious or spiritual activities, changes in belief, feelings of being abandoned or punished by God, and loss of meaning and purpose for living.

Aspects of spirituality are associated with positive outcomes, even when trauma survivors develop psychiatric difficulties such as posttraumatic stress disorder (PTSD) or depression. Research also indicates that healthy spirituality is often associated with lower levels of symptoms and clinical problems in some trauma populations. For example, anger, rage, and a desire for revenge following trauma may be tempered by forgiveness, spiritual beliefs, or spiritual practices.

Suggestions have been made about the pathways by which spirituality might affect the recovery trajectory for survivors of traumatic events. Spirituality may improve posttrauma outcomes through: reduction of behavioral risks through healthy religious lifestyles (e.g., less drinking or smoking), expanded social support through involvement in spiritual communities, enhancement of coping skills and helpful ways of understanding trauma that result in meaning-making, and physiological mechanisms such as activation of the "relaxation response" through prayer or meditation.

Feelings of isolation, loneliness, and depression related to grief and loss may be lessened by the social support of a spiritual community. Being part of a spiritual community places survivors among caring individuals who may provide encouragement and emotional support, as well as possible instrumental support in the form of physical or even financial assistance in times of trouble.

What Issues Most Often Involve Spirituality?

Making Meaning Of The Trauma Experience

Spiritual beliefs may influence the trauma survivor's ability to make meaning out of the trauma experience. In turn, the meaning drawn can have a significant impact on the survivor's symptoms and functioning. Several studies have indicated that negative thoughts or attributions about God, such as "God has abandoned me," and "God is punishing me," or, being angry at God are associated with a number of poor clinical outcomes. Research suggests that these types of thoughts can be associated with poorer physical and mental health, and increased use of substances.

Recovery of meaning in life may be achieved through changed ways of thinking, involvement in meaningful activities, or through rituals experienced as part of religious or spiritual involvement. Some researchers have suggested that traumatic events frequently challenge one's core beliefs about safety, self-worth, and the meaning of life. For individuals whose core values are spiritually grounded, traumatic events may give rise to questions about the fundamental nature of the relationship between the creator and humankind. Survivors may question their belief in a loving, all-powerful God when the innocent are subjected to traumatic victimization. In this way, traumatic experiences may become a starting point for discussion of the many ways in which survivors define what it is to have "faith."

Grief And Bereavement

Grief and loss can be significant issues that survivors must cope with in the aftermath of trauma. In U.S. society, spirituality is frequently utilized to cope with traumatic death and loss. Researchers noted after the 9/11 terrorist attacks that 90 percent of respondents reported turning to "prayer, religion, or spiritual feelings" as a coping mechanism. In general, research suggests there is a positive association between spirituality and grief recovery for survivors of traumatic loss. Researchers suggest that for many spirituality provides a frame through which survivors can "make sense" of the loss. Additionally survivors may benefit from supportive relationships often provided by spiritual communities.

Chapter 58

Laughter

There are many ways to be or stay emotionally healthy: sleep, healthy diet, exercise, etc. However, sometimes a good laugh can help us take a mental vacation from life's problems and gain some perspective. Aside from the little mental break we get, laughter is good for many other aspects of our lives.

Laughter Is A Prescription Free Medicine For Our Bodies And Minds!

Nothing works faster or is more reliable in bringing your mind and body back into balance than a good laugh. Here are some health benefits of laughter:

- Laughter relaxes the whole body. A good, hearty laugh relieves physical tension and stress, leaving your muscles relaxed for up to 45 minutes after.

- Laughter boosts the immune system. Laughter decreases stress hormones and increases immune cells and infection-fighting antibodies, thus improving your resistance to disease.

- Laughter triggers the release of endorphins, the body's natural feel-good chemicals. Endorphins promote an overall sense of wellbeing and can even temporarily relieve pain.

- Laughter protects the heart. Laughter improves the function of blood vessels and increases blood flow, which can help protect you against a heart attack and other cardio-vascular problems.

About This Chapter: This chapter includes text excerpted from "Laughter Is Important For Wellness," U.S. Department of Veterans Affairs (VA), May 12, 2015.

Laughter And Humor Help You Stay Emotionally Healthy!

Laughter makes you feel good. And the good feeling that you get when you laugh remains with you even after the laughter subsides.

- Laughter dissolves distressing emotions. You can't feel anxious, angry, or sad when you're laughing.

- Laughter helps you relax and recharge. It reduces stress and increases energy, enabling you to stay focused and accomplish more.

- Humor shifts perspective, allowing you to see situations in a more realistic, less threatening light. A humorous perspective creates psychological distance, which can help you avoid feeling overwhelmed.

Make Time To Laugh

A growing number of healthcare professionals are saying that a laugh a day may help keep the doctor away! Yes, you read that correctly—humor and laughter can cause a domino effect of joy and delight, as well as set off a number of positive health benefits.

- A good laugh can help:
- Reduce stress
- Boost immune system
- Lower blood pressure
- Lower blood glucose levels in people with type 2 diabetes
- Protect the heart
- Elevate mood

In addition, laughing can even help you lose weight! Laughing out loud for 10-15 minutes a day burns 10-40 calories, depending on a person's body weight. This translates to laughing away about four pounds a year, and every bit counts!

(Source: "Stress And Time Management," Centers for Disease Control and Prevention (CDC).)

Bring More Laughter And Fun Into Your Life!

Here are some ways to start:

- Smile. Smiling is the beginning of laughter. Like laughter, it's contagious. Pioneers in "laugh therapy," find it's possible to laugh without even experiencing a funny event. The same holds for smiling. When you look at someone or see something even mildly pleasing, practice smiling.

- Count your blessings. Literally make a list. The simple act of considering the good things in your life will distance you from negative thoughts that are a barrier to humor and laughter. When you're in a state of sadness, you have further to travel to get to humor and laughter.

- When you hear laughter, move toward it. Sometimes humor and laughter are private, a shared joke among a small group, but usually not. More often, people are very happy to share something funny because it gives them an opportunity to laugh again and feed off the humor you find in it. When you hear laughter, seek it out and ask, "What's funny?"

- Spend time with fun, playful people. These are people who laugh easily–both at themselves and at life's absurdities–and who routinely find the humor in everyday events. Their playful point of view and laughter are contagious.

- Bring humor into conversations. Ask people, "What's the funniest thing that happened to you today? This week? In your life?"

Today is a great way to start laughing. You can never be too young or too old to enjoy a good laugh. So, find a comic you like, see a comedy movie, tell some jokes with friends, anything you have to do to get out there and laugh, go do it!

Chapter 59

Interacting With Pets

Human-Animal Bond

Many people intuitively believe that they and others derive health benefits from relationships with their animal companions, and numerous scientific studies performed over the past 25 years support this belief. Among other benefits, animals have been demonstrated to improve human cardio-vascular health, reduce stress, decrease loneliness and depression, and facilitate social interactions among people who choose to have pets. Additionally, many terminally ill, pregnant, or immunocompromised people are urged to relinquish their animal companions due to concerns about zoonosis (diseases that may be transmitted between humans and nonhuman animals). However, giving up their beloved friends may have a detrimental, rather than beneficial, effect on their overall health. In many instances, human health professionals can contribute to the welfare of their patients by encouraging them to maintain bonds with their pets, even in the face of serious illnesses and other challenges.

Physiological Benefits

Numerous studies highlight physiologic benefits. Pet interaction, whether active or passive, tends to lower anxiety levels in subjects, and thus decrease the onset, severity, or progression of stress-related conditions. Furthermore, it is thought that the reduction in blood pressure achieved through dog ownership can be equal to the reduction achieved by changing to a low salt diet or cutting down on alcohol. Pet ownership and other animal contact, such as petting

About This Chapter: Text beginning with the heading "Human-Animal Bond" is excerpted from "The Health Benefits Of Companion Animals," National Park Service (NPS), February 17, 2017; Text beginning with the heading "Mental Well-Being" is excerpted from "Pets Promote Public Health!" U.S. Public Health Service Commissioned Corps (PHSCC), U.S. Department of Health and Human Services (HHS), May 4, 2015.

animals and watching fish in an aquarium, have specifically been demonstrated to provide cardiovascular benefits. Examples include:

- Increased survival time after myocardial infarction for dog owners.

- Decreased risk factors for cardiovascular disease, particularly lower systolic blood pressure, plasma cholesterol, and plasma triglycerides.

- Decreased heart rate from petting a dog or watching fish in an aquarium

These beneficial effects of pets may be mediated by increased exercise associated with pet ownership as well as decreased stress levels.

In addition to providing cardiovascular benefits, decreased physiological stress is associated with animal interaction, contributing to better overall health:

- Greater reduction of cardiovascular stress response in the presence of a dog in comparison to friends or spouses.

- Decreased pulse rate, increased skin temperature, and decreased muscle tension in elderly people watching an aquarium.

- Enhanced hormone levels of dopamine and endorphins associated with happiness and well-being and decreased levels of cortisol, a stress hormone, following a quiet 30-minute session of interacting with a dog.

- Reduced levels of the stress hormone cortisol in healthcare professionals after as little as 5 minutes interacting with a therapy dog.

Other studies document that children exposed to pets in early life experience enhanced immune function:

- Fewer allergies and less wheezing and asthma in children exposed to pets during infancy.

- Protection against adult asthma and allergies in adults at age 28 when exposed to pets before 18.

Several studies document overall general health benefits of pet ownership and animal interaction:

- Less frequent illness and less susceptibility to upper respiratory infection related to a significant increase in 18 IgA (Immunoglobulin A) levels occurred after petting a dog.

- Increased lung function and overall quality of life in lung transplant patients who are allowed to have a pet.

- Perceived pain significantly reduced in children undergoing major operations after participation in pet therapy programs.

- A significant reduction in minor health problems for at least 10 months after acquiring a dog.

- Fewer doctor visits per year for elderly dog owners than nonowners.

Companion animals have been shown to provide valuable physiological, psychological, and social benefits. These benefits are often especially significant in vulnerable individuals. Because many individuals who visit healthcare professionals are especially sensitive due to illness and the effects illness can have on one's quality of life, it is important for healthcare professionals to support the vital role of animal companionship in their patients' lives.

Psychological Benefits

Many studies have addressed the contribution of pets to human psychological well-being. One general study found that Australian cat owners scored better on psychological health ratings than did nonowners. Other studies have been more specific, focusing on groups facing stressful life events such as bereavement, illness, and homelessness. Findings from these studies often indicate that pets play a significant supportive role, reducing depression and loneliness and providing companionship and a need for responsibility.

One group of studies, performed with recently bereaved elderly subjects, demonstrated that:

- Recently widowed women who owned pets experienced significantly fewer symptoms of physical and psychological disease and reported lower medication use than widows who did not own pets.

- In bereaved elderly subjects with few social confidants, pet ownership and strong attachment were associated with less depression.

Another group of studies, looking at AIDS patients, found that:

- Patients with AIDS reported that their pets provided companionship and support, reduced stress, and provided a sense of purpose.

- Patients with AIDS reported that cats were an important part of a support system to prevent loneliness.

- Patients with AIDS who owned pets, especially those with few confidants, reported less depression and other benefits compared to those who did not have pets.

A third group of studies, carried out using homeless subjects, showed that:

- Homeless pet owners that were attached to their pets, often reported that their relationships with their pets were their only relationships, and most would not live in housing that would not allow pets.

- Over 40 percent of homeless adolescents reported that their dogs were a main means of coping with loneliness.

Studies focused on service dogs have shown overall improved quality of life for their human companions:

- Mobility-impaired individuals indicated increased "freedom to be capable" since receiving an assistance dog. Participants additionally reported increased independence and self-esteem, decreased loneliness, and experienced frequent friendliness from strangers.

- Quality of life improved in families of epileptic children when a dog that responds to seizures is present in the home.

Psychological studies reviewing the relationship between animals and children have revealed:

- The mere presence of animals positively alters children's attitudes about themselves and increases their ability to relate to others.

- Pets help children develop in various areas including love, attachment, and comfort; sensorimotor and nonverbal learning; responsibility, nurturance, and competence; learning about the life cycle; therapeutic benefits; and nurturing humanness, ecological awareness, and ethical responsibilities.

- Children exhibited a more playful mood, were more focused, and were more aware of their social environments when in the presence of a therapy dog.

Additional studies have shown:

- Alzheimer disease patients still living at home with pets had fewer mood disorders and fewer episodes of aggression and anxiety than did nonpet owners.

- Female pet-owners that have suffered physical abuse report their pets are an important source of emotional support.

- Dog owners were found to be as emotionally close to their dogs as they were their closest family members.

- Psychiatric disability patients who participated in a 10 week horseback riding program had increased self-esteem and an augmented sense of self-efficacy.

Social Benefits

Animals often serve to facilitate social interactions between people. For individuals with visible disabilities who may frequently be socially avoided by others, and in settings such as nursing homes, the role of animals as social catalysts is especially important.

- One study found that elderly people who live in mobile homes and walk their dogs in the area had more conversations focused in the present rather than in the past than those people who walked without their dogs.

- Disabled individuals in wheelchairs accompanied by service dogs during shopping trips received a median of eight friendly approaches from strangers, versus only one approach on trips without a dog.

- Observations of passersby encountering persons in wheelchairs revealed that passersby smiled and conversed more when a service dog was present.

In addition to acting as social catalysts, service dogs provide obvious practical benefits such as alerting their owners to visual hazards, auditory warnings, and impending seizures; assisting with mobility; and seeking help in emergencies. However, studies also indicate that they promote improved psychological well-being and reduce the number of assistance hours required by disabled owners.

Mental Well-Being

- Companion animals improve mental and emotional well-being in humans.

- Pet owners are less likely to suffer from stress, anxiety, and depression than nonpet owners.

- Pet therapy improves a wide array of mental health disabilities, including anxiety, panic, posttraumatic stress, mood obsessive-compulsive, and other disorders.

Obesity Preventions

- The National Institutes of Health (NIH) found that dog owners who walk their dogs are significantly more likely to meet physical activity guidelines are less likely to be obese than nondog owners or walkers.

- By providing motivation and social support, pets make it easier for owners to adopt long-term behavior changes that lead to weight loss and other positive health outcomes.

- Pet ownership is associated with key indicators of cardiovascular health such as lower blood pressure, cholesterol, and triglycerides.

Tobacco Cessation

- 28.4 percent of smokers said knowing the adverse impact of cigarette smoke on pet health would motivate them to stop smoking. Secondhand smoke exposure is associated with certain cancers in cats and dogs, allergies in dogs, and eye, skin, and respiratory diseases in birds.

Art Therapies

What Is Art Therapy?

Art therapy is based on the idea that the creative process of art making is healing and life enhancing, and is a form of nonverbal communication of thoughts and feelings. Art therapy encourages personal growth, increases self-understanding and assists in emotional reparation.

Different Forms Of Art Therapy

The spectrum of art therapy range from "Art as Therapy," where the focus is on the product (arts and crafts). The art making is used as an outlet for creative expression. At the other end of the spectrum, "Art in Therapy" is used as a vehicle for communication (psychotherapy) for the purpose of developing insight and for resolving emotional conflict.

> ### What Different Things Can Be Done?
> Drawing, painting, ceramic mold pouring, clay hand-building, wheel-thrown pottery, collage, mixed media, beadwork, polymer clay work, leather craft, pyrography, mosaics, and mask-making.

About This Chapter: Text under the heading "What Is Art Therapy?" is excerpted from "What Is Art Therapy?" U.S. Department of Veterans Affairs (VA), April 11, 2017; Text beginning with the heading "Different Forms Of Art Therapy" is excerpted from "Milwaukee VA Medical Center—Art Therapy," U.S. Department of Veterans Affairs (VA), June 9, 2015; Text under the heading "Benefits Of Art Therapy" is excerpted from "Art Therapy Provides Lifeline For Wounded Warriors," U.S. Department of Defense (DoD), November 12, 2015; Text under the heading "Music Therapy" is excerpted from "Strike A Chord For Health—Music Matters For Body And Mind," *NIH News in Health*, National Institutes of Health (NIH), January 2010. Reviewed October 2017; Text under the heading "Creative Arts Therapists" is excerpted from "Rehabilitation And Prosthetic Services," U.S. Department of Veterans Affairs (VA), January 20, 2016.

Importance Of Art Therapy

Art therapy can be used to treat and assess anxiety, depression, PTSD, substance abuse, addictions, trauma and loss, and other mental and emotional problems. It has the power to tap into unconscious material and gain access to emotions and experiences that are buried deep in the brain, without overwhelming the artist. Art therapy provides a pleasurable distraction in conjunction with exposure to difficult content so traumatic that the material can be processed.

The pleasure of creating builds self-esteem, can reduce emotional numbness, and help re-establish social functioning. In the end, the art piece can serve as a visual record and evidence of one's mental state, but it can also serve as a container for difficult emotions. Art therapy can offer solace from physical pain and relief from symptoms.

In group art therapy, one-third of the session is art making, the last third is discussion or sharing of the artwork. No one is ever forced to talk. However, reflecting on your finished piece can create new understanding and heighten self-awareness.

Benefits Of Art Therapy

Studies show creating art can produce calming effects on invisible wounds, the invisible wounds can lead to feelings of shame, guilt and identity crises that might cause them to retreat and engage in isolating behaviors. Art therapy can decrease stress hormones, which can relax and lessen anxiety—especially for those used to high-stress environments. Creating art to express feelings and help them externalize what they might have repressed for a long time can help return an affected person to a normal existence.

Music Therapy

Music can lift you up. It can bring tears to your eyes. It can help you relax or make you get up and dance. You probably hear it several times a day—on the radio or TV, in the supermarket, at the gym or hummed by a passerby. Music's been with us since ancient times, and it's part of every known culture. Music strikes a chord with all of us.

There's something about music and engaging in musical activities that appears to be very stimulating for the brain and body. Singing favorite songs with family and friends, playing in a band or dancing to music can also help you bond with others. It's a way of synchronizing groups of people and engaging in a common activity that everyone can do at the same time.

Several well-controlled studies have found that listening to music can alleviate pain or reduce the need for pain medications. Other research suggests that music can benefit heart disease patients by reducing their blood pressure, heart rate, and anxiety. Music therapy has also been shown to lift the spirits of patients with depression. Making music yourself—either playing instruments or singing—can have therapeutic effects as well.

Scientists have long known that when music and other sounds enter the ear, they're converted to electrical signals. The signals travel up the auditory nerve to the brain's auditory cortex, which processes sound. From there, the brain's responses to music become much more complex.

Over the past decade, new brain imaging techniques have shown that music activates many unexpected brain regions. It can turn on areas involved in emotion and memory. It can also activate the brain's motor regions, which prepare for and coordinate physical movement.

One brain area that's drawn interest in recent years is the medial prefrontal cortex, located just behind the eyes. In a study, this region seems to be a central hub linking music, memories, and emotion. An imaging technique called fMRI was used to look at the brains of young adults while they listened to snippets of songs from their childhoods. When they heard familiar songs, the medial prefrontal cortex lit up. Activation was strongest when the song evoked a specific memory or emotion.

"It turns out that the medial prefrontal cortex is also one of the last brain regions to deteriorate in Alzheimer disease. This may help explain why many Alzheimer disease patients can remember and sing along to tunes from their youth when other memories are lost.

Creative Arts Therapists

Creative arts therapists are human service professionals who use arts modalities and creative processes to promote wellness, alleviate pain and stress, while offering unique opportunities for interaction. Each creative arts therapy discipline has its own set of professional standards and requisite qualifications. Creative arts therapists are highly skilled, credentialed professionals having completed extensive coursework and clinical training.

Treatment Planning

Qualified creative arts therapists develop treatment goals, provide interventions, document progress, and participate as members of the interdisciplinary team. Therapists plan and carry out treatment programs that are directed to such goals as sensory integration; ambulation; diminishing emotional stress; community re-entry; reality orientation; muscular dysfunction reorientation; treatment of psychosocial dysfunction; providing a sense of achievement and progress; and channeling energies into acceptable forms of behavior.

Creative arts therapies further help patients to increase motivation to become engaged in treatment, provide emotional support for victims and their families, and create an outlet for expression of feelings. Research results and clinical experiences attest to the viability of creative arts therapies, and often for those who are resistive to other treatment approaches.

Creative arts therapists utilize a wide range of techniques of clinical interventions in applying the healing potential and influence of the arts on behavior and quality of life.

Creative arts therapists create nonthreatening group and individual art experiences for the exploration of feelings and therapeutic issues, such as self-esteem or personal insight for those with mental health needs. For Alzheimer disease, interventions are used to trigger short- and long-term memory, decrease agitation, and enhance reality orientation.

Art Therapy Has Calming Effects

Studies show creating art can produce calming effects on invisible wounds, because art therapy can decrease stress hormones, which can relax and lessen anxiety—especially for those used to staying hypervigilant in high-stress environments, Woodson said. Creating art to express feelings and help them externalize what they might have repressed for a long time can help return service members to a normal existence, he added.

Because of what they've experienced, service members often deal with a complex set of feelings and emotions that make it difficult to relate to people, Woodson said. The invisible wounds can lead to feelings of shame, guilt and identity crises that might cause them to retreat and engage in isolating behaviors," he added.

"Art therapy is a lifeline out of that isolation," the assistant secretary said.

(Source: "Art Therapy Provides Lifeline For Wounded Warriors," Department of Defense (DoD).)

Therapeutic Interventions

Interventions are used for persons with chronic illnesses to distract them from pain and facilitate needed relaxation. Creative arts therapists organize groups using art experiences to encourage self-expression, communication and socialization, and to facilitate cognitive retraining for Veterans with traumatic brain injury. The use of art-based techniques to break through barriers to the recovery process is utilized in substance abuse.

Chapter 61

Health Benefits Of Journaling

Journaling is a practice that offers significant benefits for both mental and physical well-being. It can be used effectively to handle stress, sharpen focus, and possibly even improve symptoms of illness. Journaling is known to have been practiced by heads of state, authors, and intellectuals, whose success and fame could, at least in part, be attributed to this practice.

The Benefits Of Journaling

Journaling is the act of writing down experiences in your life, as well as thoughts and observations about your feelings. This is slightly different from diary writing, which involves simply noting the events that happen in a day. Journaling as a therapeutic practice requires the capturing of one's thoughts and feelings in detail. As you journal, you develop a narrative of what events happened and then analyze why they happened and what you could have done to prevent any resulting unfavorable emotions. Through this technique, you may eventually be able to let go of emotionally debilitating feelings. Therefore, keeping a journal fulfills two main objectives: recording what happened and then learning from it.

It is often difficult to reconcile traumatic and challenging events when they occur. There's a lot to do during the course of a day, and you can't possibly stop to analyze everything that happens and why. Once something upsetting occurs, it can lead to negative thoughts, anxiety, and distress. Writing a journal for a few minutes a day provides the opportunity to think about events, describe them, and examine the emotions, thoughts, and feelings you were undergoing as they occurred and afterwards. This can help you understand your true feelings and make positive changes to your thought processes.

About This Chapter: "Health Benefits Of Journaling," © 2018 Omnigraphics. Reviewed October 2017.

Journaling can be used to educate yourself about what happened and understand how changing your thoughts and behavior can create a positive experience. Writing down exactly how you feel and identifying lessons that you've learned can help you isolate the positive aspects of events. And that can be a way of developing alternate, more productive, ways of reacting to stress and handling relationships and people.

Your journal becomes a record of how you behave and react emotionally. Regular journaling can help you manage your feelings and possibly change how you respond in the future to events that are out of your control. Journaling can help people better understand their thoughts and feelings, promote more positive ways of thinking, and help with mental-health challenges. Maintaining a journal contributes to improvement in mood, better memory, creativity, and self-awareness.

The healing power of journaling does not lie in the act of writing but in the mind. This is why psychologists believe in tapping into the power of journaling for psychotherapy. One strategy employed by some therapists is to have patients email them between sessions whenever anxiety strikes. The therapist can then provide feedback on the writing and track the patient's thinking process.

How To Journal

It is important to commit to journaling on a regular basis and devote at least 20 minutes per day to the task. Write in a place where you will be undisturbed by phones or other electronic devices. For journaling to be effective, avoid simply recounting the events of the day. Instead, write about something that is bothering you. This could be an incident at the workplace, a disagreement with family or friends, or something that is very important to you. Write about the thoughts and emotions you are experiencing related to these events. Connect the incident to your current relationships, and examine how it affects you as a person. It is possible that you may continue to write about the same event or incident for a few days, but it's best not to keep rehashing a single event for several weeks. This is especially true if you are journaling about a highly emotional incident, such as past trauma, since you may find it difficult to deal with the powerful emotions surrounding the experience.

While journaling is an excellent way to work out problems and sort out the negative feelings associated with them, it's important to capture positive, uplifting thoughts and events, as well. Many mental-health professionals suggest including things that made you laugh, incidents that made you feel grateful, and people whose company you enjoyed in your journal. You can also include challenges you overcame successfully and other activities that made you feel good. Writing down these positive feelings and events can help you find ways to repeat them.

What Does Research Say About The Benefits Of Journaling?

Various forms of writing have been used successfully in therapy for many years. Various studies have indicated that writing about emotions can also have physical benefits, such as improving the functioning of the immune system in people with physical illness. Researchers are only beginning to understand how writing is able to provide health benefits. The mere act of writing about emotions does not relieve stress. The key to the effectiveness of journaling lies in the way people interpret their experiences through writing. The use of certain types of words and phrases to express feelings seems to have an effect, as well. Journaling can help people structure and organize their anxious thoughts and reduce intrusive and negative feelings related to unpleasant events. The enlightenment that people gain from journaling is often comparable to a therapy session.

The quality of writing directly correlates to the effect it has on health. People who relive upsetting events by journaling without focusing on their underlying meaning report poorer health than those who derive meaning from the writing process. Writing with meaning helps them develop a better understanding of the emotional aspects of stressful events. Recounting events repeatedly does not relieve stress. The relief occurs when there is a change in how people perceive their experiences.

Not everyone responds the same way to journaling. People who are very reserved about their feelings tend to benefit very well from the experience. Personal qualities, such as the ability to cope with stress, self-regulate, and the quality of interpersonal relationships, are other factors that seem to determine the effectiveness of journaling.

Some researchers feel that therapeutic journaling could even help in the treatment of chronically ill people. Journal writing is, in fact, a tool with immense potential at the disposal of clinical professionals.

References

1. "The Benefits Of Journaling," University of Wisconsin Hospitals and Clinics Authority, April 13, 2016.

2. "Journaling," Regents of the University of Michigan, n.d.

3. Murray, Bridget. "Writing To Heal," American Psychological Association, June 2002.

4. Purcell, Maud, LCSW, CEAP. "The Health Benefits Of Journaling," Psychcentral. com, July 17, 2016.

5. "Writing For Mental Health," American Psychiatric Association, September 22, 2016.

Part Six
If You Need More Information

Chapter 62

Directory Of Stress And Stress Management Resources

Government Agencies That Provide Information About Stress-Related Disorders

Agency for Healthcare Research and Quality (AHRQ)

Office of Communications and Knowledge Transfer
5600 Fishers Ln.
Seventh Fl.
Rockville, MD 20857
Phone: 301-427-1364
Website: www.ahrq.gov

Centers for Disease Control and Prevention (CDC)

1600 Clifton Rd.
Atlanta, GA 30329-4027
Toll-Free: 800-CDC-INFO (800-232-4636)
Phone: 404-639-3311
Toll-Free TTY: 888-232-6348
Website: www.cdc.gov

Healthfinder®

National Health Information Center (NHIC)
1101 Wootton Pkwy
Rockville, MD 20852
Website: www.healthfinder.gov
E-mail: healthfinder@hhs.gov

National Cancer Institute (NCI)

Public Inquiries Office
9609 Medical Center Dr.
Bethesda, MD 20892-9760
Toll-Free: 800-4-CANCER (800-422-6237)
Website: www.cancer.gov
E-mail: cancergovstaff@mail.nih.gov

About This Chapter: Resources in this chapter were compiled from several sources deemed reliable; all contact information was verified and updated in October 2017.

National Center for Complementary and Integrative Health (NCCIH)

9000 Rockville Pike
Bethesda, MD 20892
Toll-Free: 888-644-6226
Toll-Free TTY: 866-464-3615
Website: www.nccih.nih.gov/tools/contact.htm

National Institute of Allergy and Infectious Diseases (NIAID)

5601 Fishers Ln.
MSC 9806
Bethesda, MD 20892-9806
Toll-Free: 866-284-4107
Phone: 301-496-5717
TDD: 800-877-8339
Fax: 301-402-3573
Website: www.niaid.nih.gov
E-mail: ocpostoffice@niaid.nih.gov

National Institute of Arthritis and Musculoskeletal and Skin Diseases (NIAMS)

1 AMS Cir.
Bethesda, MD 20892-3675
Toll-Free: 877-22-NIAMS (877-226-4267)
Phone: 301-495-4484
TTY: 301-565-2966
Fax: 301-718-6366
Website: www.niams.nih.gov
E-mail: NIAMSinfo@mail.nih.gov

National Institute of Diabetes and Digestive and Kidney Diseases (NIDDK)

31 Center Dr. MSC 2560
Bldg. 31 Rm. 9A06
Bethesda, MD 20892-2560
Phone: 301-496-3583
Website: www.niddk.nih.gov

National Institute of General Medical Sciences (NIGMS)

45 Center Dr.
MSC 6200
Bethesda, MD 20892-6200
Phone: 301-496-7301
Website: www.nigms.nih.gov
E-mail: info@nigms.nih.gov

National Institute of Mental Health (NIMH)

6001 Executive Blvd.
Rm. 6200 MSC 9663
Bethesda, MD 20892-9663
Toll-Free: 866-615-6464
Phone: 301-443-4513
Toll-Free TTY: 866-415-8051
TTY: 301-443-8431
Fax: 301-443-4279
Website: www.nimh.nih.gov
E-mail: nimhinfo@nih.gov

National Institute of Neurological Disorders and Stroke (NINDS)

NIH Neurological Institute
P.O. Box 5801
Bethesda, MD 20824
Toll-Free: 800-352-9424
Phone: 301-496-5751
Website: www.ninds.nih.gov/Contact-Us

National Institute on Deafness and Other Communication Disorders (NIDCD)

31 Center Dr.
MSC 2320
Bethesda, MD 20892-2320
Toll-Free: 800-241-1044
Phone: 301-827-8183
TTY: 800-241-1055
Fax: 301-402-0018
Website: www.nidcd.nih.gov
E-mail: nidcdinfo@nidcd.nih.gov

National Institute on Drug Abuse (NIDA)

6001 Executive Blvd.
Rm. 5213 MSC 9561
Bethesda, MD 20892-9561
Website: www.drugabuse.gov
E-mail: media@nida.nih.gov

National Institutes of Health (NIH)

9000 Rockville Pike
Bethesda, MD 20892
Phone: 301-496-4000
Website: www.nih.gov
E-mail: NIHinfo@od.nih.gov

National Science Foundation (NSF)

4201 Wilson Blvd.
Arlington, VA 22230
Toll-Free: 800-877-8339
Phone: 703-292-5111
TDD: 703-292-5090
Website: www.nsf.gov/help/contact.jsp
E-mail: info@nsf.gov

Office on Women's Health (OWH)

Office on Women's Health (OWH)
200 Independence Ave. S.W.
Rm. 712E
Washington, DC 20201
Toll-Free: 800-994-9662
Phone: 202-690-7650
Toll-Free TDD: 888-220-5446
Fax: 202-205-2631
Website: www.womenshealth.gov

Ready Campaign

FEMA/DHS
500 C St. SW
Washington, DC 20472
Toll-Free: 800-621-FEMA (800-621-3362)
Toll-Free TTY: 800-462-7585
Website: www.ready.gov/webform/contact-us

Substance Abuse and Mental Health Services Administration (SAMHSA)

5600 Fishers Ln.
Rockville, MD 20857
Toll-Free: 877-SAMHSA-7 (877-726-4727)
Toll-Free TDD: 800-487-4889
Website: www.samhsa.gov

StopBullying.gov

U.S. Department of Health and Human Services
200 Independence Ave. S.W.
Washington, DC 20201
Toll-Free: 800-273-TALK (800-273-8255)
Website: www.stopbullying.gov

U.S. Department of Education (ED)
400 Maryland Ave. S.W.
Washington, DC 20202
Toll-Free: 800-USA-LEARN (800-872-5327)
Website: www2.ed.gov/about/contacts/gen/index.html?src=ft

U.S. Department of Health and Human Services (HHS)
200 Independence Ave. S.W.
Washington, DC 20201
Toll-Free: 877-696-6775
Website: www.hhs.gov

U.S. Department of Veterans Affairs (VA)
810 Vermont Ave. N.W.
Washington, DC 20420
Toll-Free: 800-827-1000
Website: www.va.gov

U.S. Food and Drug Administration (FDA)
10903 New Hampshire Ave.
Silver Spring, MD 20993
Toll-Free: 888-INFO-FDA (888-463-6332)
Website: www.fda.gov

U.S. National Library of Medicine (NLM)
8600 Rockville Pike
Bethesda, MD 20894
Toll-Free: 888-FIND-NLM (888-346-3656)
Phone: 301-594-5983
Toll-Free TDD: 800-735-2258
Fax: 301-402-1384
Website: www.nlm.nih.gov
E-mail: custserv@nlm.nih.gov

Private Agencies That Provide Information About Stress-Related Disorders

Al-Anon Family Group Headquarters, Inc
1600 Corporate Landing Pkwy
Virginia Beach, VA 23454-5617
Phone: 757-563-1600
Fax: 757-563-1656
Website: www.al-anon.org/contact-us
Email: wso@al-anon.org

Alzheimer's Association
225 N. Michigan Ave.
17th Fl.
Chicago, IL 60601-7633
Toll-Free: 800-272-3900
Phone: 312-335-8700
TDD: 312-335-5886
Fax: 866-699-1246
Website: www.alz.org/contact_us.asp

American Academy of Allergy, Asthma, and Immunology (AAAAI)

555 E. Wells St.
Ste. 1100
Milwaukee, WI 53202-3823
Phone: 414-272-6071
Website: www.aaaai.org/global/contact-us

American Academy of Child and Adolescent Psychiatry (AACAP)

3615 Wisconsin Ave. N.W.
Washington, DC 20016-3007
Phone: 202-966-7300
Fax: 202-464-0131
Website: www.aacap.org/AACAP/About_
AACAP/Contact.aspx

American Academy of Dermatology (AAD)

P.O. Box 4014
Schaumburg, IL 60618-4014
Toll-Free: 866-503-SKIN (866-503-7546)
Phone: 847-240-1280
Fax: 847-240-1859
Website: www.aad.org/about/contact

American Academy of Experts in Traumatic Stress

203 Deer Rd.
Ronkonkoma, NY 11779
Phone: 631-543-2217
Fax: 631-543-6977
Website: www.aaets.org/contactus.htm
E-mail: info@aaets.org

American Academy of Family Physicians (AAFP)

11400 Tomahawk Creek Pkwy
Leawood, KS 66211-2680
Toll-Free: 800-274-2237
Phone: 913-906-6000
Fax: 913-906-6075
Website: www.aafp.org
E-mail: aafp@aafp.org

American Academy of Neurology (AAN)

201 Chicago Ave.
Minneapolis, MN 55415
Toll-Free: 800-879-1960
Phone: 612-928-6000
Fax: 612-454-2746
Website: www.aan.com/contact-aan
E-mail: memberservices@aan.com

American Academy of Pediatrics (AAP)

141 N.W. Pt. Blvd.
Elk Grove Village, IL 60007-1098
Toll-Free: 800-433-9016
Phone: 847-434-4000
Fax: 847-434-8000
Website: www.aap.org/en-us/Pages/
Contact.aspx
E-mail: kidsdocs@aap.org

American Association for Geriatric Psychiatry (AAGP)

6728 Old McLean Village Dr.
McLean, VA 22101
Phone: 703-556-9222
Fax: 703-556-8729
Website: www.aagponline.org
E-mail: main@aagponline.org

American Association of Suicidology (AAS)

5221 Wisconsin Ave. N.W.
Washington, DC 20015
Toll-Free: 800-273-TALK (800-273-8255)
Phone: 202-237-2280
Fax: 202-237-2282
Website: www.suicidology.org

American Counseling Association (ACA)

6101 Stevenson Ave., Ste. 600
Alexandria, VA 22304
Toll-Free: 800-347-6647
Phone: 703-823-9800
Toll-Free Fax: 800-473-2329
Website: www.counseling.org/about-us/contact-us
E-mail: webmaster@counseling.org

American Foundation for Suicide Prevention (AFSP)

120 Wall St.
29th Fl.
New York, NY 10005
Toll-Free: 888-333-AFSP (888-333-2377)
Phone: 212-363-3500
Fax: 212-363-6237
Website: www.afsp.org/about-afsp/contact
E-mail: info@afsp.org

American Group Psychotherapy Association (AGPA)

25 E. 21st St.
Sixth Fl.
New York, NY 10010
Phone: 212-477-2677
Fax: 212-979-6627
Website: www.agpa.org/contact-us
E-mail: info@agpa.org

American Heart Association

7272 Greenville Ave.
Dallas, TX 75231
Toll-Free: 800-AHA-USA (800-242-8721)
Website: www.heart.org/HEARTORG

American Institute of Stress

6387 Camp Bowie Blvd.
Ste. B-334
Fort Worth, TX 76116
Phone: 682-239-6823
Fax: 817-394-0593
Website: www.stress.org
E-mail: info@stress.org

American Massage Therapy Association

500 Davis St.
Ste. 900
Evanston, IL 60201-4695
Toll-Free: 877-905-0577
Phone: 847-864-0123
Fax: 847-864-5196
Website: www.amtamassage.org/forms/contact-AMTA.aspx
E-mail: info@amtamassage.org

American Medical Association (AMA)

AMA Plaza
330 N. Wabash Ave.
Ste. 39300
Chicago, IL 60611-5885
Toll-Free: 800-621-8335
Website: www.ama-assn.org/eform/submit/contact-us

American Meditation Institute

60 Garner Rd.
P.O. Box 430
Averill Park, NY 12018
Phone/Fax: 518-674-8714
Website: www.americanmeditation.org/
contact-us
E-mail: ami@americanmeditation.org

American Pain Society

8735 W. Higgins Rd.
Ste. 300
Chicago, IL 60631
Phone: 847-375-4715
Fax: 866-574-2654
Website: www.americanpainsociety.org
E-mail: iinfo@americanpainsociety.org

American Psychiatric Association (APA)

1000 Wilson Blvd.
Ste. 1825
Arlington, VA 22209
Toll-Free: 888-357-7924
Phone: 703-907-7300
Website: www.psych.org
E-mail: apa@psych.org

American Psychological Association (APA)

750 First St. N.E.
Washington, DC 20002-4242
Toll-Free: 800-374-2721
Phone: 202-336-5500
TDD/TTY: 202-336-6123
Website: www.apa.org
E-mail: public.affairs@apa.org

Anxiety and Depression Association of America (ADAA)

8701 Georgia Ave.
Ste. 412
Silver Spring, MD 20910
Phone: 240-485-1001
Fax: 240-485-1035
Website: www.adaa.org/contact-adaa
E-mail: information@adaa.org

Anxiety Disorders Association of America (ADAA)

8701 Georgia Ave.
Ste. 412
Silver Spring, MD 20910
Phone: 240-485-1001
Fax: 240-485-1035
Website: www.adaa.org/contact-adaa
E-mail: information@adaa.org

Association for Applied Psychophysiology and Biofeedback (AAPB)

10200 W. 44th Ave.
Ste. 304
Wheat Ridge, CO 80033
Toll-Free: 800-477-8892
Phone: 303-422-8436
Website: www.aapb.org/i4a/pages/index.
cfm?pageid=3290
E-mail: info@aapb.org

Association for Behavioral and Cognitive Therapies (ABCT)
305 Seventh Ave.
16th Fl.
New York, NY 10001
Phone: 212-647-1890
Fax: 212-647-1865
Website: www.abct.org/
About/?m=mAbout&fa=ContactUs
E-mail: clinical.dir@abct.org

Brain & Behavior Research Foundation
90 Park Ave.
16th Fl.
New York, NY 10016
Toll-Free: 800-829-8289
Phone: 646-681-4888
Website: www.bbrfoundation.org/contact
E-mail: info@bbrfoundation.org

Brain Injury Association of America (BIAA)
1608 Spring Hill Rd.
Ste. 110
Vienna, VA 22182
Toll-Free: 800-444-6443
Phone: 703-761-0750
Fax: 703-761-0755
Website: www.biausa.org
E-mail: braininjuryinfo@biausa.org

Brain Trauma Foundation
1 Bdwy.
Sixth Fl.
New York, NY 10004
Phone: 212-772-0608
Fax: 212-772-0357
Website: www.braintrauma.org
E-mail: braininjuryinfo@biausa.org

Caring.com
2600 S. El Camino Real
Ste. 300
San Mateo, CA 94403
Toll-Free: 800-973-1540
Phone: 650-312-7100
Website: www.caring.com/about/contact

Center for Young Women's Health
333 Longwood Ave.
Fifth Fl.
Boston, MA 02115
Phone: 617-355-2994
Fax: 617-730-0186
Website: www.youngwomenshealth.org/
contact-us
E-mail: cywh@childrens.harvard.edu

Cleveland Clinic
9500 Euclid Ave.
Cleveland, OH 44195
Toll-Free: 800-223-2273
Website: www.my.clevelandclinic.org

The Dana Foundation
505 Fifth Ave.
Sixth Fl.
New York, NY 10017
Phone: 212-223-4040
Fax: 212-317-8721
Website: www.dana.org/About/Contact_Us
E-mail: danainfo@dana.org

Davis Phinney Foundation

4730 Table Mesa Dr.
Ste. J-200
Boulder, CO 80305
Toll-Free: 866-358-0285
Phone: 303-733-3340
Fax: 303-733-3350
Website: www.davisphinneyfoundation.org/
contact-us
E-mail: contact@dpf.org

Depressed Anonymous (DA)

P.O. Box 17414
Louisville, KY 40214
Phone: 502-569-1989
Website: www.depressedanon.com
E-mail: depanon@netpenny.net

Depression and Bipolar Support Alliance (DBSA)

55 E. Jackson Blvd.
Ste. 490
Chicago, IL 60604
Toll-Free: 800-826-3632
Fax: 312-642-7243
Website: www.dbsalliance.org
E-mail: info@dbsalliance.org

Families for Depression Awareness

395 Totten Pond Rd.
Ste. 404
Waltham, MA 02451
Phone: 781-890-0220
Fax: 781-890-2411
Website: www.familyaware.org/contact-us
E-mail: info@familyaware.org

Family Caregiver Alliance (FCA)

235 Montgomery St.
Ste. 950
San Francisco, CA 94104
Toll-Free: 800-445-8106
Phone: 415-434-3388
Website: www.caregiver.org/contact

Geriatric Mental Health Foundation (GMHF)

6728 Old McLean Village Dr.
McLean, VA 22101
Phone: 703-556-9222
Fax: 703-556-8729
Website: www.gmhfonline.org
E-mail: web@GMHFonline.org

HealthyChildren.org

The American Academy of Pediatrics
141 N.W. Pt. Blvd.
Elk Grove Village, IL 60007-1098
Phone: 847-434-4000
Fax: 847-434-8000
Website: www.healthychildren.org/english/
pages/contact-us.aspx
E-mail: info@healthychildren.org

Hospice Foundation of America

1707 L St. N.W.
Ste. 220
Washington, DC 20036
Toll-Free: 800-854-3402
Phone: 202-457-5811
Fax: 202-457-5815
Website: www.hospicefoundation.org/
Contact-HFA
E-mail: info@hospicefoundation.org

International Foundation for Research and Education on Depression

P.O. Box 17598
Baltimore, MD 21297-1598
Fax: 443-782-0739
Website: www.ifred.org
E-mail: info@ifred.org

International OCD Foundation, Inc.

P.O. Box 961029
Boston, MA 02196
Phone: 617-973-5801
Fax: 617-973-5803
Website: www.iocdf.org/about/contact-us
E-mail: info@iocdf.org

International Society for Traumatic Stress Studies

111 Deer Lake Rd.
Ste. 100
Deerfield, IL 60015
Phone: 847-480-9028
Fax: 847-480-9282
Website: www.istss.org
E-mail: istss@istss.org

Lewy Body Dementia Association (LBDA)

912 Killian Hill Rd. S.W.
Lilburn, GA 30047
Toll-Free: 800-539-9767
Phone: 404-975-2322
Fax: 480-422-5434
Website: www.lbda.org/contact
E-mail: lbda@lbda.org

Meals on Wheels America

1550 Crystal Dr.
Ste. 1004
Arlington, VA 22202
Toll-Free: 888-998-6325
Fax: 703-548-5274
Website: www.mealsonwheelsamerica.org

Mental Health America (MHA)

500 Montgomery St.
Ste. 820
Alexandria, VA 22314
Toll-Free: 800-969-6642
Phone: 703-684-7722
Fax: 703-684-5968
Website: www.mentalhealthamerica.net/contact-us

Mental Health Minute

Website: www.mentalhealthminute.info

N. American Spine Society (NASS)

7075 Veterans Blvd.
Burr Ridge, IL 60527
Toll-Free: 866-960-6277
Phone: 630-230-3600
Fax: 630-230-3700
Website: www.knowyourback.org/KnowYourBack/Resources/KYBContactUs.aspx

National Academy of Elder Law Attorneys (NAELA)
1577 Spring Hill Rd., Ste. 310
Vienna, VA 22182
Phone: 703-942-5711
Fax: 703-563-9504
Website: www.naela.org/Web/About/
ImportTemp/About_NAELA_New.
aspx?hkey=feb0efd3-bd62-4508-9ca4-
20de373d4784
E-mail: naela@naela.org

National Alliance for Caregiving (NAC)
4720 Montgomery Ln., Ste. 205
Bethesda, MD 20814
Phone: 301-718-8444
Fax: 301-951-9067
Website: www.caregiving.org
E-mail: info@caregiving.org

National Alliance on Mental Illness (NAMI)
3803 N. Fairfax Dr.
Ste. 100
Arlington, VA 22203
Toll-Free: 800-950-6264
Phone: 703-524-7600
Fax: 703-524-9094
Website: www.nami.org

National Association of Anorexia Nervosa and Associated Disorders (ANAD)
220 N. Green St.
Chicago, IL 60607
Phone: 630-577-1330
Fax: 630-577-1333
Website: www.anad.org
E-mail: hello@anad.org

National Association of School Psychologists (NASP)
4340 E. W. Hwy
Ste. 402
Bethesda, MD 20814
Toll-Free: 866-331-NASP (866-331-6277)
Phone: 301-657-0270
Fax: 301-657-0275
Website: www.apps.nasponline.org/about-
nasp/contact-us.aspx

National Center for Victims of Crime
2000 M St. N.W., Ste. 480
Washington, DC 20036
Phone: 202-467-8700
Fax: 202-467-8701
Website: www.ncvc.org
E-mail: webmaster@ncvc.org

National Council on Problem Gambling
730 11th St. N.W., Ste. 601
Washington, DC 20001
Toll-Free: 800-522-4700
Phone: 202-547-9204
Fax: 202-547-9206
Website: www.ncpgambling.org
E-mail: ncpg@ncpgambling.org

National Eating Disorders Association (NEDA)
165 W. 46th St.
Ste. 402
New York, NY 10036
Toll-Free: 800-931-2237
Phone: 212-575-6200
Fax: 212-575-1650
Website: www.nationaleatingdisorders.org
E-mail: info@NationalEatingDisorders.org

National Eczema Society

11 Murray St.
London, NW1 9RE
Toll-Free: 800-089-1122
Phone: 207-281-3553
Website: www.eczema.org/contact-us
E-mail: helpline@eczema.org

National Federation of Families for Children's Mental Health

9605 Medical Center Dr.
Ste. 280
Rockville, MD 20850
Phone: 240-403-1901
Fax: 240-403-1909
Website: www.ffcmh.org
E-mail: ffcmh@ffcmh.org

National Gerontological Nursing Association (NGNA)

121 W. State St.
Geneva, IL 60134
Phone: 630-748-4616
Website: www.ngna.org
E-mail: ngna@affinity-strategies.com

National Hospice and Palliative Care Organization (NHPCO)

1731 King St.
Ste. 100
Alexandria, VA 22314
Toll-Free: 800-646-6460
Phone: 703-837-1500
Fax: 703-837-1233
Website: www.nhpco.org
E-mail: nhpco_info@nhpco.org

National Rehabilitation Information Center (NARIC)

8400 Corporate Dr.
Ste. 500
Landover, MD 20785
Toll-Free: 800-346-2742
TTY: 301-459-5984
Fax: 301-459-5984
Website: www.naric.com

National Stroke Association

9707 E. Easter Ln.
Ste. B
Centennial, CO 80112
Toll-Free: 800-STROKES (800-787-6537)
Phone: 303-649-9299
Website: www.stroke.org/webform/contact-us
E-mail: info@stroke.org

Parkinson's Disease Foundation (PDF)

1359 Bdwy.
Ste. 1509
New York, NY 10018
Toll-Free: 800-457-6676
Phone: 212-923-4700
Fax: 212-923-4778
Website: www.pdf.org/contact_us
E-mail: info@pdf.org

Parkinson's Institute and Clinical Center

675 Almanor Ave.
Sunnyvale, CA 94085-2934
Toll-Free: 800-655-2273
Phone: 408-734-2800
Fax: 408-734-8455
Website: www.thepi.org/contact-the-parkinsons-institute-and-clinical-center
E-mail: info@thepi.org

Phoenix House

Toll-Free: 888-671-9392
Website: www.phoenixhouse.org/contact-us

Postpartum Support International (PSI)

6706 S.W. 54th Ave.
Portland, OR 97219
Toll-Free: 800-944-4PPD (800-944-4773)
Phone: 503-894-9453
Fax: 503-894-9452
Website: www.postpartum.net/contact-us
E-mail: support@postpartum.net

Psych Central

55 Pleasant St.
Ste. 207
Newburyport, MA 01950
Website: www.psychcentral.com/about/feedback
E-mail: talkback@psychcentral.com

S.A.F.E. ALTERNATIVES

Toll-Free: 800-DONTCUT (800-366-8288)
Toll-Free Fax: 888-296-7988
Website: www.selfinjury.com/home/contact
E-mail: kconterio@selfinjury.com

Society of Certified Senior Advisors

720 S. Colorado Blvd.
Ste. 750 N.
Denver, CO 80246
Toll-Free: 800-653-1785
Website: www.csa.us/page/Contact
E-mail: Society@csa.us

Students Against Destructive Decisions (SADD)

255 Main St.
Marlborough, MA 01752
Toll-Free: 877-SADD-INC (877-723-3462)
Fax: 508-481-5759
Website: www.sadd.org
E-mail: info@sadd.org

Suicide Awareness Voices of Education (SAVE)

8120 Penn Ave. S.
Ste. 470
Bloomington, MN 55431
Toll-Free: 800-273-8255
Phone: 952-946-7998
Website: www.save.org/contact

Suicide Prevention Resource Center (SPRC)

Education Development Center, Inc.
43 Foundry Ave.
Waltham, MA 02453-8313
Toll-Free: 877-GET-SPRC (877-438-7772)
TTY: 617-964-5448
Website: www.sprc.org/contact-us
E-mail: info@sprc.org

United Advocates for Children and Families (UACF)

2035 Hurley Way
Ste. 290
Sacramento, CA 95825
Toll-Free: 877-ASK UACF (877-275-8223)
Phone: 916-643-1530
Fax: 916-643-1592
Website: www.uacf4hope.org

Visiting Nurses Associations of America (VNAA)

2121 Crystal Dr.
Ste. 750
Arlington, VA 22202
Toll-Free: 888-866-8773
Phone: 571-527-1520
Fax: 571-527-1521
Website: www.vnaa.org/contact-us
E-mail: vnaa@vnaa.org

Well Spouse Association

63 W. Main St.
Ste. H
Freehold, NJ 07728
Toll-Free: 800-838-0879
Phone: 732-577-8899
Fax: 732-577-8644
Website: www.wellspouse.org
E-mail: info@wellspouse.org

Chapter 63

Additional Resources About Stress And Stress Management

Other Teen Health Books from Omnigraphics

Abuse And Violence Information For Teens, Second Edition

Health Tips About The Causes And Consequences Of Abusive And Violent Behavior Including Facts About The Types Of Abuse And Violence, The Warning Signs Of Abusive And Violent Behavior, Health Concerns Of Victims, And Getting Help And Staying Safe

Alcohol Information For Teens, Fourth Edition

Health Tips About Alcohol Use, Abuse, And Dependence Including Facts About Alcohol's Effects On Mental And Physical Health, The Consequences Of Underage Drinking, And Understanding Alcoholic Family Members

Drug Information For Teens, Fourth Edition

Health Tips About The Physical And Mental Effects Of Substance Abuse Including Information About Alcohol, Tobacco, Marijuana, E-Cigarettes, Cocaine, Prescription And Over-The-Counter Drugs, Club Drugs, Hallucinogens, Heroin, Stimulants, Opiates, Steroids, And More

Eating Disorders Information For Teens, Fourth Edition

Health Tips About Anorexia, Bulimia, Binge Eating, And Body Image Disorders Including Information About Risk Factors, Prevention, Diagnosis, Treatment, Health Consequences, And Other Related Issues

---

About This Chapter: The mobile apps listed in this chapter were compiled from several sources deemed reliable. Inclusion does not constitute endorsement, and there is no implication associated with omission. All website information was verified and updated in October 2017.

Mental Health Information For Teens, Fifth Edition

Health Tips About Mental Wellness And Mental Illness Including Facts About Recognizing And Treating Mood, Anxiety, Personality, Psychotic, Behavioral, Impulse Control, And Addiction Disorders

Pregnancy Information For Teens, Third Edition

Health Tips About Teen Pregnancy And Teen Parenting Including Facts About Prenatal Care, Pregnancy Complications, Labor And Delivery, Postpartum Care, Pregnancy-Related Lifestyle Concerns, The Emotional And Legal Issues Of Teen Parenting, And More

Suicide Information For Teens, Third Edition

Health Tips About Suicide Causes And Prevention Including Facts About Depression, Risk Factors, Getting Help, Survivor Support, And More

Tobacco Information For Teens, Third Edition

Health Tips About The Hazards Of Using Cigarettes, Smokeless Tobacco, And Other Nicotine Products Including Facts About Nicotine Addiction, Nicotine Delivery Systems, Secondhand Smoke, Health Consequences Of Tobacco Use, Related Cancers, Smoking Cessation, And Tobacco Use Statistics

Mobile Apps For Stress Management

Beat Panic

This app contains a series of flashcards designed in soothing colors and texts that assist in overcoming the panic attack in a gentle calm manner.
Website: itunes.apple.com/gb/app/beat-panic/id452656397?mt=8

Breathe to Relax

This is portable stress management tool that provides detailed information on the effects of stress on the body and instructions and practice to help users learn the stress management skill called diaphragmatic breathing.
Website: www.t2health.dcoe.mil/apps/breathe2relax

iCBT

This app is designed to help its users to manage stress and anxiety.
Website: itunes.apple.com/us/app/icbt/id355021834?mt=8

MindShift

This app helps users to relax, develop more helpful ways of thinking, and identify active steps that will help to take charge of anxiety. It also includes strategies to deal with everyday anxiety.
Website: www.anxietybc.com/resources/mindshift-app

Pacifica

This app contains tools for stress and anxiety alongside a supportive community developed based on cognitive behavioral therapy and meditation.
Website: www.thinkpacifica.com

Panic Relief

This app guides a person through panic attacks and helps to overcome fear.
Website: www.cognitivetherapyapp.com

Self-Help Anxiety Management

This app is designed to help its users understand and manage anxiety.
Website: www.sam-app.org.uk

Worry Box—Anxiety Self-Help

This app is to learn to control worry and get relief from anxiety.
Website: www.excelatlife.com/apps.htm

Mood Sentry

This app designed to help porting of multiple computer based tools used to manage depression to a mobile platform.
Website: www.moodsentry.com

MoodMission

This is an evidence-based app designed to empower people to overcome low moods and anxiety by discovering new and better ways of coping.
Website: www.moodmission.com/app

Bust PTSD

This app is designed to help people who have experienced posttraumatic stress disorder or living with PTSD symptoms.
Website: www.cceipar.com/#section-app

ASK & Prevent Suicide

This app helps to learn the warning signs and how to ask if someone is considering suicide.
Website: www.mhatexas.org/find-help

HELP Prevent Suicide

This app provides easy access to crisis intervention resources, including a list of warning signs, steps on how to talk with someone in crisis, and information on national resources.
Website: www.app.staplegun.us/help_prevent_suicide

Lifebuoy

Lifebuoy is an interactive, self-help promoting app designed to assist suicide survivors as they normalize their lives after recent attempt.
Website: www.itunes.apple.com/us/app/lifebuoy-suicide-prevention/id686973252

R U Suicidal?

This is a video-based, interactive self-help tool for anyone having thoughts about suicide.
Website: www.psychappsint.com

Stress Doctor

This app contains breathing exercises for stress and a heart rate monitor to keep track of effects in real time.
Website: www.azumio.com

Suicide Lifeguard

This app is intended for anyone concerned that someone they know may be thinking of suicide. It provides information on warning signs of suicide, suicidal thoughts and/or intentions, and how to respond to them.
Website: www.mimhtraining.com/suicide-lifeguard

Suicide Safety Plan

This app provides six evidence-based tools to aid against clinical depression and negative moods on a large scale.
Website: www.moodtools.org

Index

Index

Page numbers that appear in *Italics* refer to tables or illustrations. Page numbers that have a small 'n' after the page number refer to citation information shown as Notes. Page numbers that appear in **Bold** refer to information contained in boxes within the chapters.